Jess has been a trusted guide for me as I've learned how diet affects every aspect of my health and performance. Crucially, she has helped me develop a way of eating that is baked into my lifestyle. Her approach gives no oxygen to the fads, just good fundamentals, actionable changes and consistent habits.

—**Rohan Browning,** Olympic 100m sprinter

Jess brings a rare combination of meticulous attention to detail and genuine practical application. Her depth of knowledge and insight is brought into the real world, which makes her expertise both powerful and actionable.

—**Bronte Campbell,** Olympic gold medallist
& Co-Founder Earthletica

For the Long Run cuts through the noise on wellbeing and performance. Jessica Spendlove makes a clear, compelling case: sustainable success comes from consistent daily habits, not quick fixes. Her 'daily operating system' is simple, practical and highly relevant — helping you build energy, manage stress and recover in a way that actually fits real life. What works particularly well is the focus on small, consistent improvements over drastic change. It's not about doing more, it's about doing what matters, consistently. For professionals and leaders, this is a sharp reminder that wellbeing isn't a luxury, it's a performance advantage. Concise, actionable and grounded in real-world experience, this is a timely guide to performing well without burning out.

—**Prof. Alex Christou,** Director Corporate Education,
Monash Business School

So many of us feel like we're doing everything right but still end up exhausted. This book explains why — and more importantly, what to do about it. In a world obsessed with quick fixes and extremes, Jess offers a thoughtful, evidence-based and deeply practical approach that shifts the conversation from managing time to managing energy. The result is a simple, human system built around small, consistent rhythms, not heroic bursts of effort, that helps you create consistency, build capacity and actually feel better as you perform.

—**Hugh van Cuylenburg,** author, Founding Director *The Resilience Project*, co-host *The Imperfects*

Jess knows her stuff. From elite athletes to CEOs to everyday people, she understands exactly what is required. Having worked at the highest levels of sport, she knows what works, and what doesn't, for all of us.

—**Melissa Doyle,** journalist, author & presenter

Jess was incredible in helping me understand my body and what nutrition and diet was required to fuel optimal performance. We tried many different techniques over different weeks and months to help me recover and perform for sustained success.

—**Toby Greene,** GWS Giants Captain, 2023 All Australian Captain

Having a vast breadth of knowledge is meaningless if you can't communicate it effectively. Jess has a brilliant way of enrolling both elite athletes and regular punters like me in developing better habits and making healthier choices.

—**Osher Günsberg,** TV host, author and podcast host

Jess supported me during my time at peak performance with Giants Netball, and I can honestly say I've never felt fitter, more confident or more in tune with my nutrition. Her knowledge, professionalism and attention to detail are exceptional. She's a true pro who genuinely cares about the people she works with, and she will make a real difference to your life.

—**Serena Guthrie,** performance coach

When trying to sift through the cloud of information, disinformation and nuance that comes with the complexities of human nutrition, health and performance, Jess is a shining beacon of sense, simplicity and applicability. She is a rare and valuable talent in the space and hearing her talk or reading her work over the past few years always leaves me better informed and more sure of my way forward. From the busy executive to the tired parent we all need a clear operating system and Jess is just the person to help us discover it.

—**Tristan Harris,** NonExec Director, former CoCEO and former Chair Harris Farm Markets

Over the past few years, I've seen different waves of modern wellbeing. It's an overwhelming landscape, full of big promises and unrealistic overhauls that are hard to sustain. *For the Long Run* offers a refreshingly practical alternative. It meets you where you are, helping you build on what you're already doing rather than demanding a complete reinvention of your life. Well researched and highly actionable, Jessica's warm and at times fun tone makes it genuinely accessible, it offers thoughtful guidance that feels both empowering and achievable. Her concept of a daily operating system just makes sense. It's simple, effective, and easy to apply.

I found myself making small, meaningful changes straight away. Even something as simple as upgrading a meal that same day. Recommended reading to anyone looking to live and perform better and who's tried and failed at all the fads!

—**Barbara Harvey,** Head of Learning Growth Faculty

Jessica Spendlove has distilled years of elite performance experience into a practical, intelligent system for real life. *For the Long Run* unlocks high performance for every human, one practical habit and small shift at a time. It closes the gap between knowing what to do and actually doing it, with simple, sustainable habits that protect your energy and elevate your performance over time. This is the kind of framework every high performer needs on their desk.

—**Shannah Kennedy,** high performance life coach and author of *The Life Plan*

Jess has had a profound impact on my longevity in the AFL. She has a rare ability to translate complex nutrition principles into simple, sustainable and flexible practices. Most importantly, she challenged many of my long-held beliefs in a way that has reshaped my thinking and unlocked a whole new level of performance.

—**Dane Rampe,** Sydney Swans AFL player, Co-Captain 2019–2023

For the Long Run is a really practical book to optimise your health, particularly if you're a high achiever. Jess's focus on progress not perfection makes it much easier to adopt her strategies.

—**Adjunct Prof. Sophie Scott OAM,** health communications expert

I saw Jess Spendlove speak at an event and her no-nonsense approach to life choices had an immediate, material impact on me. As entrepreneurs and business owners, we can't pour from an empty cup — this is a marathon, not a sprint. Business leaders need all the help they can get. *For the Long Run* gives us exactly what we need: practical, science-backed tools to look after ourselves so we can sustain the performance that matters most.

—**Naomi Simson,** OAM, business leader, entrepreneur, speaker

FOR THE LONG RUN

FOR THE LONG RUN

Build your **daily operating system** for **energy, recovery** and **wellbeing**

JESSICA SPENDLOVE

WILEY

First published 2026 by John Wiley & Sons Australia, Ltd

ISBN: 978-1-394-43465-7

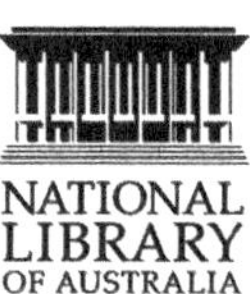

A catalogue record for this book is available from the National Library of Australia

Registered Office
John Wiley & Sons Australia, Ltd. Level 4, 600 Bourke Street, Melbourne, VIC 3000, Australia

For details of our global editorial offices, customer services, and more information about Wiley products visit us at www.wiley.com.

Wiley also publishes its books in a variety of electronic formats and by print-on-demand. Some content that appears in standard print versions of this book may not be available in other formats.

Cover design by Wiley
Cover image: © mstMazeda/stock.adobe.com

Set in 11/16pts and Palatino LT Std by Straive, Chennai, India.

For Millie

Thank you for putting everything into perspective.

For you

Thank you for being here.

My hope is that these pages challenge you to think differently about performance, recovery and success, and to see your wellbeing as the foundation for everything.

I hope this book offers a way forward that is evidence based, but also designed to fit your life. Because when that happens, you elevate your wellbeing and sustain your performance, now and for the long run.

Contents

About Jessica Spendlove

Jess Spendlove has built her career at the intersection of wellbeing and high performance.

She is an international speaker, podcast host and advisor who has spent more than 15 years helping ambitious individuals and teams achieve sustainable performance.

Jess holds a Bachelor of Science in Nutrition and a Master of Nutrition and Dietetics. Through her involvement with elite sport, corporate leadership and the military, she has worked inside some of the most demanding performance environments in the country, gaining a rare perspective on what it truly takes to sustain success under pressure.

A former national swimming champion, Jess went on to build and lead performance nutrition programs across seven professional Australian sporting teams with the GWS Giants AFL and AFLW, Cronulla Sharks, Sydney Kings, Giants Netball, NSW Waratahs and Western Sydney Wanderers. She worked alongside Olympic medallists and premiership-winning teams and has advised the ADF School of Special Operations for the last seven years.

Her individual clients have included James Magnussen, Rohan Browning, Errol Gulden and Dane Rampe.

Today, she works with leaders, teams and organisations to turn wellbeing into a performance and leadership edge through her keynotes, workshops and strategic programs. She is an associate with Monash Business School's Corporate Education Program. In recent years, her work has evolved beyond nutrition. Jess now focuses on the broader architecture of sustainable performance, translating elite principles into everyday strategies and systems that keep people sharp, healthy and performing well at work and in life. She shares these insights through her work and each week on her podcast, *Stay at the Top*.

Jess has not just studied wellbeing and performance, she has lived it. From elite sport to supporting top performers in business, high-growth start-ups and the military, and now navigating life as a new mum, she understands that wellbeing evolves across seasons. Having witnessed the cost of neglecting it, she is committed to reshaping the narrative, so success is achieved because of wellbeing, not at its expense.

Jess lives in Sydney with her daughter Millie and partner Sam.

How to use this book

This book is designed to be read in order. Each chapter builds on the one before it, creating a clear and practical pathway for elevating your wellbeing and sustaining performance. While some sections may feel more immediately relevant to you, the real power comes from understanding how the pieces connect and compound.

You do not need to implement everything at once. In fact, I would encourage you not to. Sustainable performance is built through upgrades, not overhauls. Read with curiosity, reflect on what resonates and identify one or two strategies to upgrade, tweak or strengthen before moving on.

You may return to different chapters at different stages of your life or career. What feels most important now may shift over time. That is normal. Your health is not something you set and forget. Wellbeing evolves across seasons.

This book is not about perfection. It is about building the foundations that allow you to perform, recover and lead well in work and life, now and for the long run.

Introduction

Do you ever feel like you're doing most things right, yet you're still exhausted, overwhelmed and constantly on the back foot?

Maybe your energy is inconsistent. You never feel fully recovered. And despite your best efforts, you still can't fit as much into your day as you'd like.

I hear this all the time—and from people you'd probably be surprised to hear it from: CEOs to unicorn founders, Olympic medallists, world champions, premiership-winning athletes, special forces operators and everyday people juggling work, family and life.

While their lives and pressures may be different, they have a similar story: 'I feel like I'm doing most things right, but…'

For over 15 years I've worked at the intersection of wellbeing and high performance. I've supported hundreds of elite athletes; built and run the performance nutrition program for seven professional Australian sports teams; consulted inside military and special operations environments; advised leadership teams; spoken to groups of senior executives and CEOs; and coached high-performing individuals who are driven, capable and deeply committed to doing their best.

After all of that, what I have learnt is this.

Most people understand the basics in theory—eat well, sleep well, move often—and they think they are doing an okay job at these things. But when we dive a little deeper below the surface-level knowledge, the issue usually comes down to one of a few things.

They struggle with consistency, they live reactively rather than proactively and they prioritise everyone and everything before themselves—their children, their career, their teams, their business. Sound familiar?

When this is happening, of course your energy will be flat or inconsistent, or you'll never feel fully recovered. You cannot keep putting yourself last and expecting your body to keep delivering.

Usually, there is more context too. A busy thriving career; ever-evolving hybrid work, which has been great for flexibility but has also disrupted any sense of routine; young children, families or ageing parents, all of which mean more logistics. Frequent bouts of illness across the year (which always seem to hit at the most inconvenient times) leave you thinking: *Why does it always happen like this?*

This is where most people go wrong. They jump to the conclusion that the solution is something drastic. They just need to 'kick start' or 'reset' things with a six-week challenge or a four-day juice cleanse or a three-day water fast. Eenie, meeny, miney … *no!*

The secret sauce to elevating your wellbeing and performance today, tomorrow and in the future is finding your own definition of *consistency*. Consistency you can implement when routines are disrupted, work is demanding, children are sick and energy is low.

Please don't think that when I say consistency, I mean rigidity and that you need to eat the same thing every day or commit to a seven-day-a-week gym routine. I don't. I can set the record straight on this now. That is not the solution.

This book is not about doing more, it is about doing what actually matters in a way that fits your real life. Much of what we focus on here is not about adding new behaviours but upgrading the ones you are already doing every single day, things like what you eat and how you sleep. The great news is that it's generally easier to upgrade or tweak something you're already doing than add something new.

You'll also learn how and why you should work with your biology. Despite all the advancements in tools and technology we've had, our human biology has not changed for thousands of years, so learning to leverage this and live more in alignment with it presents a huge opportunity.

This book will show you how to build a daily operating system that brings structure to your health, energy and wellbeing, so you are no longer guessing, reacting or constantly resetting. An operating system can help you create more sustainable energy rather than chase it, recover before you are depleted or need to take burnout leave, and build the capacity to handle the pressure and stresses that you're faced with day after day.

There are three questions you will be able to answer clearly by the end of this book:

- How do I create and sustain energy?
- How do I manage stress and build my tolerance to it?
- How do I recover more effectively?

The goal is to help you perform well now, feel better in your body and mind, and apply strategies that work with where you are starting from, while also building habits and systems that still support you five, ten and 20 years from now. Sound like a plan?

Your health — now and in the future

The future of your health is determined by the daily decisions you make like what you eat, how you move your body, how you manage your stress, how you sleep and how connected you are to your purpose and the people who matter.

These daily decisions shape how much energy you have, how well you recover and how you show up each day. They also compound over time, quietly and powerfully, influencing not just how you feel this week or this year, but the quality of your health, wellbeing and performance for decades to come.

These are the foundations to your wellbeing and sustainable performance. They are made up of the behaviours that move the needle both now and in the future, and they are where your attention needs to be focused first, to find consistency and rhythm.

In this book, you will learn practical tools, strategies and ways of thinking that help you create, optimise and sustain energy; recover more effectively; and build the capacity and stress tolerance required to perform in a demanding, fast-paced world. Most importantly, you will learn how to do this in a way that actually works for your life, not someone else's version of a ten-step, 5 am routine you feel like you should be following. Phew!

What you can expect

Let me ask you something. Would you prefer to have good health now or in the future as you age? I don't know about you, but I would like option C please. *Both!*

The strategies in this book are designed to improve the quality of your life today: to give you more consistent energy, to have you feeling more recovered, and like you have more capacity to handle what life throws at you. They are also built with the long game in mind—to protect and extend not just your lifespan, but your health span.

The decisions you make today do not just affect how you feel in the short term. They accumulate and compound. They shape the trajectory of your health, your energy and your ability to perform over time. This is why this book is about the long run.

The long run is how you run your life, day after day, using the daily operating system you build through your routines, behaviours and rhythms. When these are intentional, proactive and customised to your life, they support your energy, recovery and capacity today, while also setting you up for your future.

This book is about elevating how you feel every single day, while knowing you are paying dividends to the future version of yourself. That is what it means to build wellbeing and sustainable performance *for the long run*.

Foundations over fads

The ideas in this book are not theoretical. They are grounded in physiology, behavioural science and years of real-world application. They reflect patterns I have observed repeatedly across elite sport, military environments and corporate leadership teams over the past 15 years.

While the contexts and pressures differ, there are the same breakdowns with energy, recovery and stress when the foundations are not consistently prioritised. There are also huge improvements when simple, well-structured habits and systems are put in place.

We live in an information economy. Podcasts, social media, wearables, AI and an endless stream of expert opinions have given us unprecedented access to health advice. And yet, despite knowing more than ever, we are more confused, more exhausted and more burnt out than ever before.[1,2]

At the same time, the future of health is genuinely exciting. It is personalised, customised and data driven. If you are reading this book, chances are you already engage with health information. You listen to the podcasts (hopefully mine). You follow your trusted experts. You are exposed regularly to new protocols, trends and tools through social and mainstream media alike.

The ice baths, the red-light therapy, the endless list of supplements—or are we meant to be doing the IV vitamin infusions now?

Don't get me wrong, some of these tools may have a place. In the right context, for the right person, at the right time, they may offer some gains. But when they become the focus at the expense of the foundations, they distract from what actually drives energy, recovery and performance, both now and in the future.

I am sorry to say you cannot ice bath your way out of chronic sleep debt, or IV vitamin infusion your way out of a poor diet. Someone needed to say it!

As the information economy has grown, I have also noticed another problem alongside confusion. Fatigue from constant decision-making.

We've been left feeling like we need to be doing everything all at once. Like we're meant to follow every protocol, optimise every metric, and apply the ten-step 5 am protocol that works for our favourite podcast host. A protocol that recommends you run a marathon, read a book, have an ice bath, journal—all before getting to work. Okay, that might be a slight over-exaggeration, but you get my point.

We're exhausting ourselves before the day has even begun.

When health behaviours are not built on strong foundations, implemented consistently and tailored to our lives, they become forced. They demand too much push energy and mental bandwidth to maintain, and they simply become unsustainable.

Marginal gains

The real leverage lies in upgrading what you are already doing. This mirrors the concept of marginal gains, also known as the 1% improvement principle, popularised by Sir Dave Brailsford during his time as performance director of British Cycling. While that team, era and some practices have since come under scrutiny and been debated, the principle itself has stood the test of time and proven more durable than any one team's story.

At its core, it's about breaking performance into its smallest components and improving each one incrementally. Over time, the cumulative effect of those incremental improvements becomes transformational.

We see this approach across many industries, from elite sport to medicine and business. When small, deliberate improvements are applied across multiple areas, the combined impact outperforms any single overhaul.

In elite sport, areas to make adjustments include recovery, nutrition, sleep, psychology, environments and systems. Sound like your life? It should.

This framework and philosophy isn't reserved only for athletes or sports teams. It is exactly how sustainable high performance in life is achieved. Not through one dramatic change, but through hundreds of small, deliberate upgrades layered onto what already exists. Nothing is too small to matter.

This idea is echoed by James Clear in *Atomic Habits*, where he writes:

> *It is so easy to overestimate the importance of one defining moment and underestimate the value of making small improvements on a daily basis … Improving by 1 percent isn't particularly notable—sometimes it isn't even noticeable—but it can be far more meaningful, especially in the long run.*[4]

From a behavioural and biological perspective, this is how humans change best. Small upgrades to existing behaviours are far easier to sustain than complete overhauls because they work with established routines, neural pathways and environmental cues, rather than against them. Yet, in practice, this is rarely how people approach changes, particularly when it comes to their health and performance. The temptation to overhaul everything and chase fast results is strong, and it often drives all-or-nothing behaviour.

When you take a different approach and adjust just one or two behaviours at a time, change becomes manageable. You create space to notice what is working, and just as importantly, how it feels. This is a principle we will return to throughout the book.

The path of least resistance

I also believe we have been sold a lie when it comes to health: the lie that it must be hard, that progress requires constant discipline, restriction and effort. The truth is that it can feel much easier than this, but only when the approach meets you where you are and helps you choose the path of least resistance rather than asking you to fight your life at every turn.

This approach also trains you to notice the green flags. The subtle signals that tell you when something is working. Signals like more stable energy, better focus, improved sleep, less road rage. These are often missed when you are trying to change everything at once.

When you stop attempting to overhaul your entire life and instead make small, intentional adjustments to what you are already doing, the process changes entirely.

This is where the idea of a daily operating system emerged. Not as another set of strict rules or exact protocols to follow, but to organise behaviours around purpose and rhythms.

There are five rhythms that make up your daily operating system. These are your:

1. nutrition: what you eat and how you fuel your body each day
2. exercise: when you move your body and the type of movement you do
3. stress and recovery: how you deliberately downshift and recover from stress across your day, week and year
4. sleep: how you support regular, restorative sleep through timing, routine and environment
5. connection: how you maintain connection to purpose, people and the things that matter most.

For many of us, knowing what to do is rarely the problem. The issue becomes applying this knowledge consistently in a way that works for our lives, and understanding how these behaviours can fit and be customised to our lives, rather than forcing what works for someone else.

What helps sustain behaviour change is understanding why those behaviours matter, and how they fit within the broader demands of your life. This is where the daily operating system comes in.

Daily operating system

At its core, your daily operating system serves a few key purposes. It helps you get clear on what is important to your health, it is tailored and customised to you, and it helps you attach the behaviours in it to a key function. Ultimately, it is designed to give you clarity, structure and flexibility, all of which are important.

The purpose of the operating system is to provide:

- clarity on where you should focus your energy and efforts rather than feeling like you need to piecemeal it together
- structure, with a road map and framework that provide a process you can follow
- flexibility with a variety of inputs, meaning you can select which ones speak to you or feel like the path of least resistance to apply.

All three of these are equally important to your long-term success of consistently being able to sustain any new or upgraded behaviours you implement. They also help you reframe the question from:

What should I be doing?

And help you answer this question with a lot more purpose by asking:

What is the goal of this behaviour? Why do I want to do this behaviour? What do I want to achieve with this behaviour?

There are three core functions in your daily operating system, which I classify as the three Cs. They are:

1. Charge up

This about how you create, optimise and sustain energy, and include behaviours that sit at the front of the day, as well as the rhythms you build across it to achieve elevated and more sustained energy.

2. Capacity

Here we look at how well you handle stress. Capacity reflects your ability to tolerate pressure, adapt to challenges and remain resilient over time.

3. Charge down

Just as important is recovery, not just at the end of the day, but across it. Here we focus on how you downregulate your nervous system, create space between effort and intentionally design moments and rhythms of recovery into your day and life.

Most importantly, establishing your daily operating system is about giving you a framework you can apply proactively. When you have your own operating system, it puts you in the driver's seat. This allows you to set the tone for the day rather than react to it.

Now, the most important thing to know here is that this doesn't just allow you to get back to baseline, it helps you elevate that baseline. As you start to put this into practice, in a way that works for your life and helps you live proactively, you will be surprised at the difference it makes. I am so excited for you to experience it!

The other thing for you to know is that living proactively, rather than reactively, isn't as big of a shift as it might sound. It is all about you knowing a few key non-negotiable behaviours that you can implement, not just on your best days, but on your busiest.

How I arrived here

My perspective on this work has been shaped by decades in high-performance environments, and by observing the same patterns repeat themselves. I have seen this across elite sport, military settings and corporate environments. And I have lived it myself.

For as long as I can remember, I carried a narrative that I could do more than most people. That my capacity was simply greater. Part of that came from how I was brought up. Hard work was valued. Effort was rewarded. That belief was also shaped very early through sport.

From the age of nine, I was waking at 4.15 am to swim for two hours before school, then travelling back across Sydney to train for another two hours after school. That was my normal, but it wasn't exactly the 'normal' thing every nine-year-old was doing.

By the time I was competing at a national level at age ten, that way of operating was ingrained. Doing more, training more, spending my days from 4.15 am until 8.30 pm on the move, go-go-going.

When something becomes unsustainable, whether in sport or in life, performance does not plateau, it goes backwards. I started to experience exactly that in my teens. I was getting sick more often. I felt constantly exhausted, like I was running on fumes. And yet, paradoxically, this only reinforced the belief that my capacity was higher than most people's. I started to think that operating in a state of exhaustion was normal and forgot what feeling energised at training and focused at school felt like.

That belief followed me well beyond the pool. It shaped how I studied, how I worked and how I approached my career. I said 'yes' to everything. I worked multiple casual jobs while studying. I took on more responsibility, more pressure, more load. At one point, I was working full time in a hospital, I'd started a PhD and I was working part-time in a clinic to transition my career into professional sport.

When I moved into professional sport, the pattern continued. Where most people might work with one or two teams maximum, I worked with seven—at the same time! I built a business, had a team of junior dietitians and students underneath me, and I relied heavily on my ability to push through, to do more than most people, and on the ego-driven belief that I could handle it.

What I didn't understand was this: when you operate in an unsustainable way, it is not a question of *if* things unravel, but *when*. I've had my fair share of those moments. The kind where you think, *surely, I should have got the memo by now.* Like the time I forgot my laptop was on the roof of my car and drove over it. Or the time I sent one of the most embarrassing reply-all emails of all time to the CEO of a sports team I worked with the day before our Christmas party. I got roasted all night. I am still embarrassed about it now nearly ten years later!

Here's the thing. You might be able to operate at a high level like this for many years, but, eventually, you pay the price in some way. By the time I had established my career in professional sport, and was working with multiple teams at once, I couldn't understand why I was running on fumes—looking back now, it is crystal clear.

Sure, I was eating well, I was exercising, I was sleeping fine, largely because I was exhausted. But recovery was almost non-existent. Stress was consistently high and work had become my entire life. I was working six to seven days a week for nearly the entire 12 months of the year, year after year. This included long 12- to 14-hours days and travelling around the country for games. I missed birthdays, I rarely saw friends other than my best friend who I lived with at the time when I was occasionally home, and despite doing what I loved, I started to feel empty.

Looking back, I experienced burnout on and off for four to five years straight, but it all came to a head after I had COVID-19. I spent 12 to 18 months unwell, bedbound for days and weeks on end, chasing answers. It took all of this for me to finally receive the memo: that the way I had been operating was not sustainable. This was the catalyst that set me on the path to do the work I now do and bring this work into the world.

Wellbeing and sustainable performance without an operating system is a short game, as your health is the foundation that everything is built on.

If you are reading this book, chances are you want results now, but you are also thinking about future you. You do not want to work hard today only to burn out tomorrow or not experience the joys of your hard work in decades to come. You want to build something that lasts, which is what I call *sustainable performance*, and that's what we're going to do here together.

What's ahead

The chapters that follow will help you build this operating system step by step. We begin by slowing things down and learning how to listen to what your body is already telling you, because self-awareness is the foundation of change. Next, you will learn how to work with your human biology, and find a rhythm that feels more easeful, like swimming with the current rather than against it.

From there, we work through the five key rhythms of your daily operating system: nutrition, exercise, stress and recovery, sleep and connection. We'll explore how each one helps create and sustain energy, expands your capacity and stress tolerance, or facilitates recovery more effectively. Many of these rhythms influence more than one outcome, reinforcing that health is an integrated system, not a set of isolated behaviours or silos.

Finally, we piece it all together, so you feel excited, clear and ready for your own daily operating system. We will also cover off how you can adapt it to all of life's variables, whether that is travel for work or life, or when you are navigating a different season of life.

I hope at this point you're as excited as I am to create and sustain energy more consistently, recover proactively and with intention, and expand your ability to handle pressure over time.

This is not about doing everything at once. It is about building a system that supports how you want to live, work and perform, not just on your best days, but on your busiest ones. When daily non-negotiable behaviours are applied consistently, across months and years, they compound.

In the short term, they help you show up with more energy, feel more rested and recovered, and protect your wellbeing. In the long term, they are what allow you to perform and sustain your wellbeing and success *for the long run*.

Part 1

A daily operating system for sustainable performance

Chapter One

Why you need a daily operating system

If I asked you, 'What do you need to do to prioritise your health more?', I am sure you would answer with a version of the following. I need to:

- eat more vegetables
- drink more water
- sleep eight hours a night
- exercise daily or most days
- manage my stress better.

At a high level, most of us know what supports our health and what undermines it. Eating well most of the time, moving regularly, sleeping more and staying hydrated are all correct. The question is not whether we know this, but whether we are able to execute it consistently.

If knowledge alone were enough, very few of us would struggle, which is why the issue today is not necessarily a lack of information.

The problem is the growing disconnect between what we know we should be doing and what we're able to execute consistently in our lives. This doesn't mean there aren't things to learn—there is plenty that I will share with you in this book—but the biggest problem is the ability to perform those behaviours consistently, in a way that works for your life.

We have never had more access to expert knowledge, high-quality research and credible education around health and performance than we do right now via social media and podcasts, and yet, despite this, people are not healthier. They are not more consistent. They are not finding it easier to sustain behaviours when pressure increases or routines are disrupted. This is why the conversation needs to shift not just from *what* we need to do, but to *how* we do it consistently, particularly when life is busy, unpredictable and demanding.

Declarative versus procedural knowledge

There are two different types of knowledge. Declarative knowledge is knowing *what* to do. Procedural knowledge is knowing *how* to do it in the real world. Research I did during my masters comparing elite athletes with the general population found that, in both groups, declarative knowledge is largely there. What's lacking is the skills and strategies to turn that knowledge into consistent action.[5]

This is where the idea of a daily operating system comes in.

If knowledge alone is not the problem, then something else must be missing. What is missing is a system that helps translate what you know into the behaviours you can sustain even when life puts you under pressure.

For that system to work, it cannot be generic. It must be customised and tailored to your life, your constraints and the season you are in.

One size does not fit all

I believe another reason this gap continues to widen is due to how a lot of information is presented. Health advice can be packaged and over simplified *(e.g., just follow this exact ten-step protocol).* Sure, that protocol may deliver an impact while you force it into your life, but what happens when life gets busy or you get tired and you stop or skip some of the steps?

Forcing someone else's set-and-forget protocol is like wearing a tailored suit made for another body. The materials may be high quality and the design is great, but it hasn't been fitted to you, it does not move with you and it never quite feels right. With a set-and-forget protocol, the issue is the lack of personal context and customisation. It just forces something into your life without truly understanding where you are at. This is why customisation for your life, your constraints and your starting point is such a crucial step within your operating system.

The great news is that most principles for health and wellbeing are universal. The nuance sits in the application. Of the thousands of people I have worked with, I never forced a behaviour onto someone. I start by understanding their life, their constraints, their goals and what they are currently doing, and then help tailor the principle accordingly.

Take nutrition as an example, which is the first rhythm we will cover. One principle we will explore is pulsing protein intake, spreading it more evenly across the day, with particular attention to breakfast, which is an area where many people fall short. That same principle can support a CEO wanting steadier energy, someone wanting to lose body fat and gain muscle, or an athlete looking to recover better or maximise performance.

But the application depends entirely on the individual. If someone is getting what they need some days, but not others, the focus is on how to help them adjust that. If they skip breakfast all together, the strategy will look different to someone who dabbles with fasting some days or who prefers something 'not too heavy' because they 'aren't that hungry in the morning'. Depending on where each person is starting from, the principle remains the same, but the application differs.

For the person who doesn't eat breakfast, the goal is to start having something to create the habit. For the person who is inconsistent with their breakfast, the goal is to standardise their morning more. For the person who wants something light, we might look at a protein smoothie, rather than eggs or salmon.

The principles stay the same, but the execution changes.

Hybrid work

The way many of us work has changed. Hybrid and flexible work have delivered plenty of benefits, including more autonomy and less time commuting, but it has also quietly removed many of the default rhythms and anchors that once supported more consistent behaviours.

Commute time plus office hours created a natural bookend to our days. Office-based work tended to support more consistent rhythms around meal and break times. And while fixed schedules were not perfect, they did provide clearer external cues around when work typically started or ended.

Without these cues, or by experiencing them less consistently, the lines between work and life have blurred. In the process, many of the external cues that once supported more consistent rhythms around when we eat, move, recover and switch off have been removed or become less consistent.

Why consistency is so important

Consistency does not mean doing the same thing every day or living a rigid, robotic life. It means having enough structure to support you regardless of variation, disruption or curveballs. I often think of this like bumpers in a bowling alley. They are there to stop every ball from ending up in the gutter.

This is what I believe is the sweet spot. Structure that creates stability without rigidity. Rhythms made up of behaviours that work for your life, that allow for adaptability without requiring perfection or an all-or-nothing approach. This is what I refer to as *structured flexibility*.

When we stop seeing consistency as a set of perfect conditions and see it as clarity on the behaviours that are most important to our health, energy and performance, something shifts. It becomes less about waiting for the ideal day and conditions and more about identifying the opportunities that already exist to execute those behaviours.

Consistency also matters because it allows us to leverage momentum rather than rely on willpower or motivation. Instead of deciding each day whether you feel like taking action, the decision has already been made. For example, you do not need to rely on motivation to go to the gym. In your operating system, you train three times a week. One of those sessions is on Wednesday morning, it is in your diary and your week is structured around it.

The energy lie we have all been told

Most of us believe our biggest constraint is time. If only we had more hours in our day, more space in our calendar or fewer competing demands, we would finally be able to prioritise ourselves and be more consistent with our health.

But time is not the real constraint, energy is. In a *Harvard Business Review* article, Tony Schwartz and Catherine McCarthy made the point clearly: 'time is finite, but energy can be systematically expanded and renewed'.[6]

Energy determines how you show up every day, the quality of your decisions, your emotional regulation, your patience, your focus and essentially what you can manage in your day. When energy is good and stable, we make better choices almost effortlessly. When our energy drops, our standards drop with it, and everything becomes harder and more exhausting. Under fatigue and pressure, even our good intentions become inconsistent or more unreliable.

We have been sold a lie about energy.

Energy is not something you either have or do not have. It is not about springing out of bed ready to go. It is not a personality trait or a reflection of how driven you are. Energy is something you create through the decisions you make and the systems you build every single day!

Think about your phone. If you want it at 100 per cent in the morning, you need to plug it in, give it time and avoid draining it overnight. If you forget, or only half charge it, you cannot expect it to perform the same way the next day. Your energy works the same way.

It's worth mentioning that there are different types of energy. Performance psychologist Jim Loehr described energy as multidimensional with four key aspects:

1. Physical energy determines the quantity of energy you have available, your basic capacity to meet the demands of the day.
2. Emotional energy shapes the quality of that energy, whether you operate from curiosity and challenge or from pressure, threat and frustration.
3. Mental energy directs where your energy goes, your ability to focus, prioritise and stay with what matters.
4. Spiritual energy provides the force behind it—your sense of meaning, values and why the effort is worth it.[7]

These four dimensions are interconnected. When physical energy is depleted, focus and emotional regulation suffer. When emotional energy is constantly driven by stress, mental clarity declines. When work lacks meaning, even when we are well-rested, we can struggle to sustain effort and output.

Tip: Energy and recovery are two sides of the same coin

Energy is something you create. When you identify what reliably builds your energy and you do this consistently, your energy becomes more stable and predictable.

Recovery is what allows you to repeat this day after day. It is where you reset, downregulate and recharge so your energy can be sustained. Recovery is not the opposite of performance, it is what makes consistent performance possible.

Why your body and brain need rhythm

There is a reason predictable patterns matter so much for health and performance. The body and brain function best when there is rhythm, expectation and a degree of regularity, rather than constant uncertainty or guessing. When key behaviours such as eating, movement, sleep and recovery happen at roughly the same time, energy can be directed toward thinking, decision-making, creativity and emotional regulation instead of on navigating what comes next.[8]

Chaotic days, skipped meals, sporadic recovery and inconsistent routines create subtle physiological strain over time that accumulates. The result of this? Fatigue increases, focus becomes harder to sustain and everything requires a bit more effort and energy each time.

This is why a well-designed structure feels stabilising and supportive, and provides you with more space and capacity for other things. It also reduces the number of decisions required to get through the day and lowers the energy cost of simply operating.

Predictable patterns give the body a reliable baseline to work from, even when our days and what we will be facing is unpredictable, which conserves energy and helps expand our tolerance. It makes flexibility possible without it becoming exhausting. Like an operating system, the basics are handled quietly in the background, freeing capacity for everything else.[9]

It's time to get off the reactive rat race

Do you think you live reactively or proactively? In my experience, most of us are living reactively by default. We respond to the demands of the day as they arise, make decisions on the fly and hope there will be enough left in the tank to recover later. We eat when there is a gap in our diary. We rest only when we're exhausted or sick. We skip meals or movement when we get busy and promise ourselves we will 'start again Monday' or 'tomorrow' or 'when this project is delivered'. Sound familiar?

This reactive loop is incredibly common. In the short term, it's easier to just go with the flow, but this inconsistent, reactive way of living, which is generally the result of what other people need from us at work or home, is eroding our energy and capacity and not allowing us to recover properly.

When we miss what's important for our needs, like a lunch break away from our desk with a nourishing meal, and instead replace it with something we quickly scoff down in front of our computer mid-afternoon, we are not only putting everything before ourself, but we are making small reactive decisions that are slowly compounding to leave us feeling exhausted and always behind. Additionally, when recovery is treated as a response to depletion rather than a planned investment, we spend most of our time hovering just above empty like the person who always runs their car petrol range down to the last 5 kilometres and then frantically looks for the closest petrol station.

If this all sounds familiar, there is no judgement here. Honestly, I see this pattern repeatedly in my work, and I spent years operating like this myself, so I not only help people make this switch, but I have also done this myself.

Do you know a Gary or a Sarah?

I bet you know a Gary or a Sarah. Or maybe you recognise yourself in one of them. Gary, the CFO, is brilliant, driven and consistently performing. Sarah, the COO, is equally brilliant and driven and just as impactful.

Both are high performers who carry significant responsibility. Over time, however, the difference becomes more obvious.

Gary performs without chaos. He is consistent, produces sustainably and rarely runs on fumes. Sarah still delivers, but she is often pushing too hard, running on empty and holding things together through sheer effort.

The difference between Gary and Sarah is not capability or technical expertise, it is that Gary operates proactively, and Sarah lives reactively.

Proactive living means deciding in advance how you will protect energy, rather than responding once it is already gone. Gary builds recovery and energy into his days and weeks. He does some movement each morning before he gets to work, he has a set and protected lunch break. He also has a sauna a few times a week, and he goes to a health retreat once a year—not to fix his burnout, but to stay ahead of it. Sarah on the other hand is often seen having lunch at her desk around 3 pm, if at all. Recovery only happens when her body forces her to stop and she gets sick. Eventually, she takes the burnout holiday just to reset, which really just gets her back to baseline.

The biggest gap between Gary and Sarah is a daily decision to live proactively rather than reactively. Because the truth is, every day you get to decide how you operate. This book is designed to give you the tools to choose the former.

Why the shift from reactive to proactive is so important

This is one of the most important shifts you can make. Moving from operating reactively to proactively does not require as much of a dramatic change as you might think. It begins with awareness, structure and being intentional.

This is also where most of us get stuck. We understand that energy matters, but we don't know how to consistently protect it in the context of real life because we are often benchmarking against what we can do in an ideal situation, rather than in our reality.

For too long, health and wellbeing have been framed as hard work, discipline and sacrifice. Something that must be forced, endured or squeezed in when time allows. Sustainable energy is built by choosing the path of least resistance, by aligning behaviours with biology, by creating conditions that make good decisions easier, not harder.

If energy is the true currency of health and performance, then the behaviours that create, optimise and sustain it must be intentionally designed into our day. That does not come by accident or by living reactively, it comes by being proactive. The best solution I have seen to help this switch is to have a daily operating system that adapts with life's demands.

The chapters that follow are built on this idea. Energy is not found, it is created, and creating it requires consistency and structure that allows for flexibility and adaptability, especially when life is full.

Sprint versus marathon thinking

Do you love watching the Olympics? I do! I particularly enjoy tuning in to the 100-metre sprint to see who the fastest man or woman on the planet is.

Beyond the swagger, the glitz and the glam, what really stands out is how these athletes are built. Sprinters like Noah Lyles are built for power and speed, with explosive muscles and short bursts of maximum output for a very brief window of time. Everything about a sprinter's body screams explosive power!

Now compare that with a marathon runner. They are just as impressive but built very differently. Athletes like Eliud Kipchoge are shaped by efficiency and endurance, with an ability to sustain effort for hours.

Imagine if they swapped events. How do you think Noah Lyles would go in the marathon, or Eliud Kipchoge in the 100-metre sprint? Probably not that great.

The truth is, very few people can do both well. The physical demands, energy systems, pacing strategies and recovery requirements are fundamentally different. Yet, today, we are all essentially expected to be world class at both. We are expected to sprint through our days with urgency and intensity, while also lasting the distance over the weeks, months and years.

As a result, most of us are operating in a state of always being on and always being available. We've got one hand and eye on the dinner table while we eat dinner, and the other on our phone and Slack channel. We check our inbox on the weekend while we are out to brunch with friends or family, or maybe at half-time during our kid's sport. The line between work and rest, being on and switching off, has become increasingly blurred or non-existent for many. Trust me, I get it!

For a long time, I told myself that being available 24/7 was a strength. That being constantly available to the athletes I worked with, responding to messages at any hour, made me better at my job and in demand. Those porous boundaries came at a huge cost to myself and, in particular, my health. My nervous system was constantly overstimulated, and there was no real separation between work and life—it was all one big, overstimulating, exhausting blur.

I now see the same pattern repeatedly in the work I do with leaders and leadership teams. Leader wellbeing is one of the strongest drivers of organisational wellbeing and performance.[10] When leaders operate in an always-on, reactive way, those behaviours cascade through teams. This is often referred to as the *contagion effect*. Energy, stress and behaviour spread, whether we intend them to or not. When leaders operate with clarity, intention and recovery built in, those patterns also ripple outward. When they do the opposite, the same happens.

This is why the way you operate matters, not just for you, but for the people around you: your family, your friends, your team. Without clear boundaries, there is no endpoint to effort. Your recovery is non-existent, your stress accumulates and, over time, your capacity erodes until you get rundown, burnt out or sick.

Burnout doesn't happen in one dramatic collapse, it happens through thousands of small mismatches between effort and recovery. What once felt manageable begins to feel heavy. Sure, you may continue to perform for a period of time, but it becomes increasingly exhausting or depleting. It feels like you are surviving, rather than thriving. This is the definition of death by a thousand papercuts! So many of us are operating like this.

Whether you like it or not, your daily behaviours compound and you cannot separate how you operate today from how you will feel in five years' time. The body keeps a quiet record of how often it is asked to push versus how often it is allowed to restore. And, as I learnt the hard way, operating unsustainably always comes at a cost.

One of the most useful principles I took from my time working in professional sport to help manage this is *periodisation*.

The principle of periodisation

Periodisation refers to the deliberate variation of load and recovery over time. Athletes do not train at the same intensity every day, every week or every month. Their training is structured in cycles, with different demands across days, weeks and longer phases of the year.

In team sports such as AFL, NRL, netball, basketball, rugby union or soccer, the year typically follows a clear pattern.

In pre-season, the goal is to build as much fitness and capacity as possible. The days are longer than at any other time of the year, and the training load is higher. Sessions are harder across the week, with a clear focus on developing physical fitness, strength and conditioning. This is where athletes do the work to expand what their body can tolerate later in the season.

In-season, the focus shifts to competing. Training becomes less about building and more about retaining. The priority is recovery, resilience and maintaining as much of the fitness and strength built earlier in the year as possible, while staying healthy and available to perform.

Off-season allows space for recovery and rest, without stopping altogether. Training volume and intensity come down, structure loosens, and both physical and mental fatigue are addressed. Movement continues, but in a way that restores rather than depletes, so athletes return to the next pre-season ready to build again.

In comparison, most of us operate in one mode—flat and linear at 100 per cent all the time. Every day is treated like a peak performance day. Meetings run back-to-back, stimulation is constant and daily recovery looks like Netflix on the couch while we scroll Instagram or TikTok.

The point here is not that you need to live like an athlete, but that there are lessons worth considering, such as how you can apply the principle of periodisation to your life. That might not be a day-to-day or week-to-week variation, but it might be reducing some of your commitments when you know you have a particularly demanding time at work.

A daily operating system bridges short-term performance and long-term resilience by introducing variation where life has become flat, building recovery in before depletion forces it, and allowing you to perform well today without borrowing from tomorrow. This is the shift from sprint thinking to marathon thinking.

Your daily operating system

Regardless of whether you enjoy putting together a flat pack from IKEA or not (I don't), one thing is certain—you need the instructions!

Try putting together furniture without them and you end up with spare parts, wasted time and something that never quite works the way it should. That is exactly what is happening with health and performance right now.

We are being fed one-minute reels and TikToks every day, jumping from fasting to cold exposure, to breathwork techniques, supplements and new protocols, and if you are honest with yourself, that has probably become the bulk of your research. You find yourself piecing together tactics and behaviours without any overarching system or clarity on where you should focus your time, effort and energy.

The problem (in most instances) is not the strategies themselves, it is the lack of context being provided. They don't tell you the full story or take you from start to finish when it comes to breaking down how all these strategies fit together. Just like the IKEA flat pack without instructions, this approach lacks a clear operating manual, which brings us to what I believe is the solution: creating a personal daily operating system.

This concept is not new. In fact, it already governs many other areas of your life whether you realise it or not. Your phone, computer and the systems you rely on at work all operate this way. When an operating system is working well, you barely notice it; it quietly supports performance in the background. It only becomes obvious when it becomes outdated or requires updating.

Wellbeing is no different. Most of us only realise we don't have a system that is working for us when things start to feel difficult, inconsistent or when we are trying to level up and can't seem to make it stick.

At its core, having a daily operating system for your wellbeing exists to cut through noise and complexity and helps you be clear on what you need to operate well day after day. It helps you prioritise your health first, not as a luxury, but as the foundation that allows you to show up with energy, clarity and capacity across every other area of life.

The three core functions of your daily operating system

As we touched on back on page xxvi, in the context of your health and wellbeing, your daily operating system serves three core functions:

1. *Charge up:* How you create and sustain energy across the day. A big part of this is how consistent your mornings are, and what you do across the day to top up and sustain your energy.
2. *Capacity:* How you increase your capacity and ability to operate under pressure by building your stress tolerance.
3. *Charge down:* How you recover more effectively. This is about how you end your day, and how you build moments of recovery into the day and cadences across the year.

Your operating system is designed to support your energy, your capacity and your recovery. Together, these determine how you feel and perform today, as well as in the future.

The five rhythms

The five rhythms that make up your operating system are your nutrition, exercise, stress and recovery, sleep and connection.

I use the word *rhythms* deliberately as it gives the sense of flow, consistency and repeatability rather than rigidity or perfection. Rhythms are designed to work with your life, not against it, which is why this approach often feels easier and more sustainable than what you may have tried before. Remember, this is about choosing the path of least resistance.

Together, these rhythms, and the one or more behaviours in them, make up your daily operating system. That system provides you with structure, priority and clarity around what matters most to your wellbeing. It helps you operate at your best by understanding what assists you in creating and sustaining energy, what lets you expand your capacity and resilience, and what improves your recovery.

This is also where the idea of an operating system can be misunderstood. It is not about rigidity or doing the same thing every day, in fact, the opposite is true. A daily operating system creates structure without rigidity. Most importantly, it is built for real life. Because it is adaptable, it meets you where you are, and most importantly, it is customised to *you*.

To bring this to life, here are two examples from my own daily operating system.

My exercise rhythm includes a mix of strength, cardio, walking and yoga across the week. Before having my daughter, this almost always happened in the morning, but now, that is not always possible, so I need to be more flexible. What stays consistent is that I move my body every day—even if it's just a short walk. The reason I do this is because it charges me up and helps me create and sustain energy. Other times, such as with an after-work walk, it helps me charge down from the work day. The rhythm provides structure, without locking me into one rigid way of doing things, which wouldn't work with this rhythm in this season of life. It gives me structured flexibility.

My sleep rhythm, on the other hand, is more structured. It includes consistent cues that help my body prepare to sleep. These include not drinking coffee after midday and not watching TV after 8.30 pm at night. If I am out for dinner, which doesn't happen much these days with a one-year-old, I opt for a 6 pm or 6.30 pm booking so I can still stick with the same timing and structure. Protecting my sleep is high priority, as it helps me charge down and effectively recover each night, which also largely determines what my energy is like the next day.

Your current season of life

Let me ask you an important question: are you benchmarking your health, habits and capacity against what is realistic for your life right now, or against the best you have ever been? This is a trap that can be easy to fall into, and, if I am honest, it is one I have fallen into myself recently.

After I gave birth to my daughter, I developed chronic back pain. At first, it was persistent but not that bad, and I assumed it would resolve with time and me doing the usual things like seeing a physio, getting regular massages and modifying my movement accordingly.

Instead of improving, the pain lingered and slowly worsened. After months of little progress and further investigations, including an MRI, I had to come to terms with where things were at. What I was asking of my body no longer matched the season of life I was in. Despite everything I had been doing to fix it, the pain was not improving, so something needed to change more drastically.

Part of that adjustment meant changing up the exercise I was doing and returning to the pool. Swimming and I have a complicated relationship. Years of early mornings and long sessions staring at a black line tend to do that. I am certain I reached my lifetime quota of staring at a black line in my teens.

Getting back in the water also involved overcoming plenty of mental hurdles, which included excuses like, 'Oh, I will have to wash my hair'. At first, the challenge was simply showing up. Then came the comparison against the 15-year-old version of me swimming 5 to 8 kilometres per session, eight to nine times a week—not the 38-year-old version with chronic back pain, a one-year-old, broken sleep and an entirely different set of responsibilities.

That comparison was never going to be fair or helpful. What eventually shifted was the lens I was using. I reframed what swimming meant to me, so it was no longer about performance or output, which is what my DNA always knew it as, but about movement, process and maintaining my exercise rhythm, which is important for my mood, energy and overall operating system.

I am going to be honest, consistency with exercise is never something I have struggled with until this year. The back pain was a factor. Becoming a new mum was another factor. Figuring out a way to upgrade or change my exercise rhythm to fit this current season of life, including not only what I could do, but when I could do it, was a huge factor.

I had to learn to be more flexible and, while I prefer to exercise in the morning and get it out of the way, that isn't always possible right now. I needed to upgrade my exercise rhythm to have more flexibility while retaining the structure. This was not about having unrealistic expectations of myself, it was about figuring out what mattered to me, my wellbeing and what was possible for me right now.

This is a point I often emphasise in my work: *Sustainable progress rarely comes from doing more.* It comes from reducing friction, removing extremes and designing rhythms that are centred around being consistent.

The goal is not to recreate the best you have ever been, it's to meet yourself where you are right now and build from there. When your rhythms are designed for the life you are living, not the ideal one you are benchmarking against, consistency becomes possible, and consistency, over time, is what compounds.

Lastly, the goal is not for you to do everything, it is to understand where you are, and what is realistic and sustainable. To support this, each section in this book will have an activity so you can take stock of where you are currently and start to piece together your operating system. This is a modified version of the life audit process I use with my coaching clients.

The other thing you need to know before building your operating system is what your body is already telling you. Most of us miss the early signs and only pay attention when things really get in the red or break—like me. In the next chapter, I will show you how to start listening properly, so you can build a system that fits your life as it is right now.

Activity

Take a moment to reflect on how you are currently operating by reflecting on these questions.

- How do you usually start your day? Is it consistent or does it vary? Think about behaviours like what you eat, what you drink, if you exercise.
- How do your days typically end? Do you have a consistent routine before you go to bed or does it vary? Think about your behaviours before bed and note the time you go to bed on weekdays and weekends.
- How well do you currently handle pressure? Do you feel stressed? Does it feel sustainable for the next few months or years or are you getting by week to week?

Conclusion

Creating a daily operating system is about creating structure without rigidity. When you do this, your body and brain trust what is coming next. You waste less energy navigating chaos, and you have more energy available for the things that actually matter.

Chaotic behaviours and days quietly create physiological strain, which, over time, mean everything slowly requires a bit more effort and energy.

The currency central to your health and performance is energy, and when it comes to energy, this is not something you either have or you don't. It's something you create through daily behaviours. This is what the five rhythms that make up your operating system are built on, and they support the three key functions: how you charge up and create energy, how you build capacity to manage stress, and how you charge down to recover consistently over the days, weeks and months that make up your life.

Chapter Two

It's time to learn a new language

Have you ever been to a foreign country where you don't speak the language and tried to navigate your way around with Google Translate? You usually get there in the end but it can be frustrating, clunky and everything takes longer as you're trying to figure it out.

Now compare that to travelling with someone who speaks the language fluently or, better yet, a local guide. Suddenly, everything moves faster. Decisions are easier and the overall experience is tailored. You see what matters, avoid what doesn't and may even get to skip the queue and head straight to front of the line like I did in Rome. Amazing!

This is exactly what is happening with your body and brain every single day. They are constantly communicating with you, sending updates, offering feedback, providing you with insights. The problem is that most of us have never learnt how to interpret or understand them.

Between work, family, deadlines, devices and the constant pull of external demands, these messages get drowned out. If you are honest with yourself, you probably do notice some of them: low energy, poor focus, cravings, changes in mood. Instead of listening to them or trying to interpret what they are saying, you push through or reach for a quick fix. Hello, 4 pm coffee, which you know you are going to regret later, but you do it anyway. YOLO!

When early signs and signals like these are ignored, they do not disappear. Instead, what starts as a whisper becomes a nudge. A nudge becomes a warning. Eventually, it is yelling at you, impossible to ignore, and that's when most of us, including a past version of yourself, hear them.

Learning to tune in to these signals is one of the greatest advantages you can have. This is the language of your body and brain, and it's always communicating with you. These signs and signals directly communicate how you are operating, and whether you're working with your biology or against it. In my opinion, these are far more powerful, and take a lot less of your time, than any three-hour podcast you might be listening to.

These signs and signals you're receiving are personalised data. They are your body and brain speaking to you. Likely, up until now, you just haven't understood them, had time or been able to decode them. Just like any new language, it takes time, practice and consistency to become more fluent.

This chapter is going to introduce you to this new language and then, over time, as you become more fluent with it, you'll understand more clearly what it is trying to tell you. The more obvious messages will stand out at first, but over time, even the more subtle ones will become clearer. I invite you to be curious with them, and to notice any patterns or trends that emerge.

Figure 2.1 is a visual snapshot of some of the most common signs and signals your body and brain use to communicate with you. Notice which ones you experience. Some of these may show up regularly for you, while others might occur less often. Bringing awareness to this is the first step.

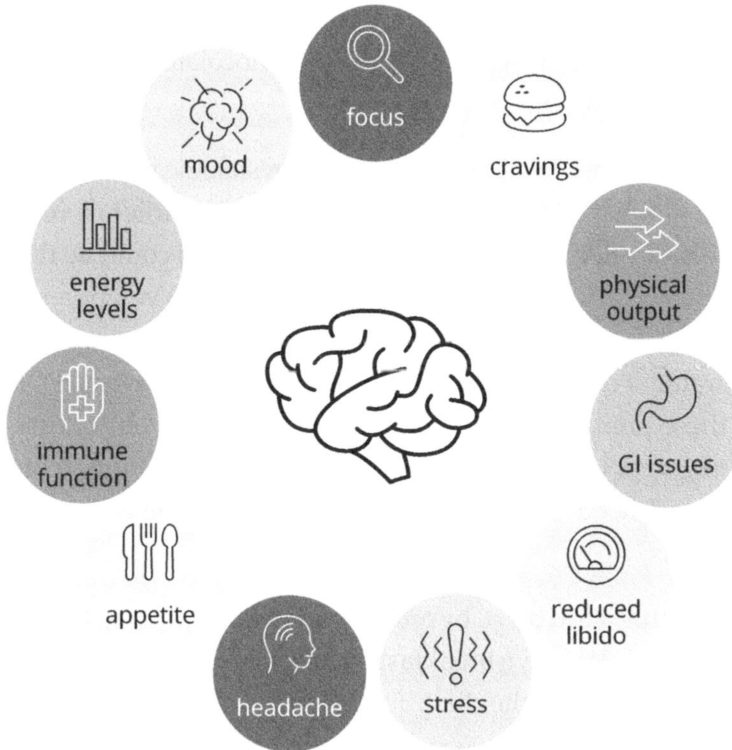

Figure 2.1 *Ways your body and brain communicate with you*

What we think our body is telling us versus what it's actually telling us

This might surprise you, but I do not believe in cravings. Well, not in the way most people think of them. In my experience, cravings are not random or a lack of discipline. They are messages that your body and brain are trying to tell you something.

Now, I am not talking about you walking past an ice-cream shop or bakery on the weekend and then deciding you want one. I am talking about the predictable cravings that hit at the same time regularly. For you it might be the 3 pm chocolate cravings, or the evening salt-and-vinegar chips.

These regular, predictable cravings are physiological. They show up because you have missed something important earlier in your day. I call this the 'flow-on effect'. What you've missed could be that you haven't eaten enough food across the day, or you've got a specific nutrition gap such as not enough protein or fibre, or maybe you're dehydrated. Potentially, it's a combination of all of these. So, if you have these predictable, regular cravings, they are your brain's way of saying to you, 'Hey, hello! You haven't given me enough of what I need, so I need that extra tasty thing to give me an immediate pick me up!'

A lot of this can be a byproduct of us living reactively and inconsistently. We have breakfast sometimes, but don't other times. We wait for a gap in the diary to eat lunch. We wait for the energy crash to happen before we reach for the coffee and whatever is on the counter. When the goal is to operate proactively, a big part of building your daily operating system is finding your definition of regularity through rhythms so your body and brain know what to expect in a predictable and consistent way.

The upside of this is huge. It not only makes life easier for you, but it elevates how you feel every single day. I am so excited for you to learn how to do this in a way that fits your life, as it makes such a huge difference to how you show up every day.

When you learn to interpret this language, you stop fighting your biology and begin working with it. To understand these signs and signals properly, it is helpful to have a daily dashboard made up of two pieces of information: subjective metrics and objective data.

> ***Tip: Subjective metrics and objective data***
>
> *Subjective metrics* tell you how you feel; for example, how rested do you feel when you wake up each morning? How consistent is that across the week?
>
> *Objective data* shows you what is happening underneath the surface with your physiology; for example, what was your total sleep time? How much time did you spend in deep and rapid eye movement (REM) sleep?

I strongly believe, the real power comes from blending both subjective metrics and objective data, as that blend is where self-awareness meets self-management. Tuning into how we feel is important for everyone, it's free and you can do it anywhere, anytime. By pairing these subjective metrics with objective data you can see exactly what is going on with your own physiology. I believe it is the combination of these two that really puts you back in the driver's seat of your health and performance.

The metrics that matter

I believe subjective metrics are the best place for you to begin, as these are intuitive and immediate. They also reveal your earliest signs of change.

Three of the most important subjective metrics are energy, appetite and performance:

1. Energy is about how much you have—your total energy levels, as well as the stability and consistency of that energy across the days, weeks and months.

2. Appetite is how hungry you are over the day. Do you arrive at meals ready to eat, or do you swing between starving and overfull? This also includes cravings, which, as mentioned, are mostly signs and avoidable. Cravings that appear consistently in the afternoon or evening are not coincidence, they are communication.
3. Performance is the most individualised metric of the three, and it includes both physical and cognitive performance. Everyone has a combination of these that matter, but they will be in different ratios depending on the demands of their day and life. For example, physical performance is more about how you move, train and how your body feels during and after effort. Cognitive performance, on the other hand, is more about your focus, your ability to concentrate and your ability to get into flow and do deep work without distraction.

Reflection: Do you have an energy gap?

If you had to rate your current energy out of ten, what would you give it? Now consider where you would ideally like it to sit. What would that be? Is there a gap?

When you start paying attention to these cues, patterns emerge. You will start to see what drains you and what restores you. You will also start to understand what lifts your performance and what undermines it.

Most importantly, you realise that energy is not fixed or something you do or don't have. It is something that is created, and future chapters will help you identify what that is for you.

Tip: Your energy shift

As you move through this book and begin making changes, pay attention to how your energy responds. It will shift in both directions depending on how well you support yourself.

This feedback is critical. It is part of the new language you are learning.

This observation is the beginning of self-awareness. It is how you start to connect your habits and behaviours to your biology, and how you start to define the behaviours that make up your five rhythms. Over time, these observations will start to feel effortless and automatic, and you will get clear on your own daily operating system.

Best of all, you will understand which behaviours and rhythms help you charge up by giving and sustaining your energy; which ones help build your resilience and stress tolerance, expanding your capacity; and which ones help you recover more effectively and charge down. This helps you get clear on what really matters and understand how specific habits and behaviours work for you or against you.

Subjective metrics tell you most of the story, but on their own, they do not always give you the full picture of what is happening under the hood from a physiology perspective. This is where objective data can add value, helping you make more informed, data-driven decisions to help you corroborate how you feel.

What is happening under the hood

There are elements of your physiology that you simply cannot reliably detect through feel alone. Changes in recovery, nervous system load, time spent in the most restorative phases of sleep, or accumulated fatigue often occur in the background before you consciously notice them via how you feel.

This is where the benefit of objective data comes in as it can give you more visibility into what is happening under the hood with your own physiology before it comes to the surface with how you subjectively feel. Objective data can show how your body is responding, adapting and recovering, not just how it feels in the moment. When subjective awareness is combined with the right objective metrics, decision-making becomes clearer, more informed and far less reactive. Let's look at a useful tool to help you measure your objective data.

Using wearables

In my opinion, this is where the use of wearables comes in. Devices such as the Oura ring or WHOOP band can provide you with access to biometric data that goes beyond a standard watch. I am, personally, a strong advocate for these wearables, not because the data is perfect, but because it gives you more visibility. It allows you to spot patterns, trends and early warning signs that are otherwise easy to miss, and to adjust before something feels off or you get rundown or sick.

If you are reading this section and noticing a sense of resistance, perhaps thinking that you don't want a wearable, don't want access to more data, or that this feels like another thing to manage, that is completely understandable. It may also be something you simply do not want to explore right now.

Nothing in this book depends on technology to work. The foundation of this approach is awareness, behaviour and biology. You can apply everything here with or without a wearable and still experience meaningful change.

If a wearable feels useful, it can support the process. If not, you are not missing out on the work that matters most. That does not mean what follows is irrelevant to you.

I intentionally began this chapter by focusing on subjective metrics, because they are available to everyone. In fact, most meaningful change shows up here, and can look like more stable energy, feeling less tired, improved focus at work, less irritability, having enough energy left at the end of the week to enjoy time with the people you care about.

Wearables can add another layer of insight by providing objective data, such as resting heart rate, heart rate variability and sleep patterns. Over time, they can help you see trends and patterns that are harder to notice day to day. That said, they are a tool, not a requirement.

If using a wearable feels helpful to you or you're open to it, the way I like to think about the data that comes from a wearable is similar to a profit-and-loss sheet for your health. It helps you keep your finger on the pulse of key information such as:

- how well you are recovering
- the quality and consistency of your sleep
- your overall stress and strain load.

It is important to be clear about what this is not. This is not about obsessing over every single metric every single day. When people fixate too closely and let the data dictate how they feel, a helpful tool can quickly become unhelpful.

In my opinion, the real value is in the history and trends you see over time. When you zoom out and use objective data as part of your broader dashboard, it adds context, it shows patterns, and this is what can really help support better and more proactive decisions.

Sometimes the data from wearables can also help reinforce progress, and who doesn't like a pat on the back? You have been getting more restorative sleep, your energy is stable, and the numbers reflect that. That feedback can be helpful, build confidence and reinforce the behaviours that have driven those outcomes.

At other times, the data highlights strain. Subtle changes in recovery, sleep or stress load can validate what you are already sensing and prompt an earlier, more informed decision.

One of my favourite points about objective data is that it gives you something to compare over time. It reveals your baseline and shows you when you are drifting away from it. That is how you detect periods of increased stress and strain early, and how you recover and bounce back faster. This includes your:

- recovery
- sleep quality
- strain
- stress load
- physiological trends.

This is how you catch problems early. This is how you adjust before you break down. This is how you protect both wellbeing and performance.

A decision-making tool

How often do you get sick at the worst possible time? Maybe for you that's right before a board meeting, a pitch, a keynote, a holiday you have been looking forward to for months. Gosh, it's so frustrating, isn't it!

I've had my own fair share of these experiences in the past and saw this clearly on a recent international keynote trip to Queenstown. My first trip since having my daughter.

It was part of a three-day summit for a group of CEOs. I had the option to fly in just for my keynote or attend the full program. I decided to go for the full program as I wanted to make the most of the experience, see the other speakers and meet as many people attending as I could.

I arrived feeling slightly off, but not enough to raise concern. My Oura ring data looked stable, but (subjectively) I felt a bit off, so I decided to rest in my room that afternoon before the first formal event later that night.

The next morning, over breakfast with a group of CEOs, I started to deteriorate quickly. I was overheating and having difficulty regulating my temperature. I returned to my room and checked my Oura ring data. There it was. Major symptom radar! Something I had never seen before.

When I dived into the metrics in more detail, there it was in black and white:

- elevated temperature
- increased respiratory rate
- dropping heart rate variability
- rising resting heart rate
- a readiness score in the 30s rather than my usual 80s or 90s.

At that point, my physiology was speaking in complete sentences. It corroborated everything I was feeling! I was not well, and I needed to take cover and rest. So, I made the call to rest for the entire day.

That was absolutely not what I wanted to do. I had not flown to another country without my baby to sit in a hotel room. I had flown there to learn, network and experience the summit. But, ultimately, the main thing I was there to do was deliver the final keynote.

If I had pushed through on day two rather than rest, I risked not being able to do the very thing I was there to do—get on stage and speak!

Reflection

Be honest with yourself, how many times can you think of where you 'pushed through' and then paid the price?

This is the power of blending subjective and objective data.

My subjective cues gave me the early signals. The objective data confirmed the severity. Together, they allowed me to make a data-driven decision that protected my performance. One without the other would have been incomplete, and I would have 100 per cent found a way to justify that 'I wasn't that bad'. I would have pushed through, and the outcome would have been catastrophic. The data made the decision that much easier.

When you combine subjective cues with objective insights, you stop guessing. You lead yourself with clarity. You stop fighting your physiology and begin working with it, and you feel less guilty for making the call to sit out the dinner or the day, because it will save you missing the entire week or, in my experience, the keynote I had flown to another country to deliver.

Now that you understand your dashboard, you are well on your way to elevating your self-awareness, which really is a true superpower.

Self-awareness is your superpower

Self-awareness is your superpower when you harness it. The important thing to understand is that it is a skill, which means it is learnable. Once you develop it, it begins to underpin every decision you make about how you work, recover and perform.

I really believe the power of self-awareness is underestimated in terms of the role it plays in driving and sustaining behaviour change. What self-awareness does is bring you back to the present. It shifts your focus from the outcome to the process. When it comes to improving health and performance, people often fixate on big goals, such as losing weight, gaining muscle, running faster, lifting heavier. These are all worthwhile goals, but slow by nature, and they involve an external measurement to determine success.

When progress takes time, it can feel like nothing is happening. Motivation drops, doubt creeps in and, as a result, goals can be abandoned because there is not enough feedback along the way.

This is the downside of being overly outcome focused. Outcomes, like weight loss, take time to show up. For some, when those markers do not move quickly enough, it is easy to jump to the conclusion that what we are doing isn't working, and we lose momentum and interest.

When the lens shifts from the outcome to the process, behaviour change becomes easier to sustain. Instead of focusing on weight loss, the focus becomes energy, consistency and how you feel day to day. These are immediate signals that are directly linked to the behaviours that drive the long-term results you are seeking. Ironically, by tracking what you can notice and influence daily, you are more likely to stay consistent long enough to reach the outcome you are chasing in the first place.

This is where I like to introduce the idea of green flags. You may be familiar with Matthew McConaughey's book *Greenlights*, which reflects on moments that moved him forward in life. Green flags are similar, but they're about noticing in real time.

Green flags

Green flags are the small, often uncelebrated signals that tell you you're on the right track. They include:

- more stable energy across the day
- better focus in the morning
- fewer cravings in the afternoon
- improved sleep quality
- training that feels strong and like you can go to another gear
- a sense that you are coping better, even when life is full
- getting sick less often than you normally do across winter
- having more energy on the weekend for friends, family or activities you love.

These green flags show up in behaviour and how you feel long before the outcome you are chasing does. When you learn to recognise them, you stop measuring progress only by distant results and start reinforcing the daily process that creates change, and celebrate the small but significant wins along the way.

One of the core ideas I want to reinforce throughout this book is that *consistency beats intensity*. Most of us already understand this in other areas of our lives, even if we do not consciously think about it that way. Investing is a good example. We know to be wary of get-rich-quick schemes as they rarely work, but what does work is regular contributions, patience and time in the market. The same is true for superannuation, where small, consistent deposits quietly compound over decades.

Yet, when it comes to health, that logic often disappears. We can be so tempted to reach for the quick fixes: the six-week challenges, the four-day detoxes, the extreme resets, the promise of a clean slate on Monday or a fresh start in the new year. Yet, the reality is, it has taken a lifetime of habits to get you to this point. You can't expect to 'reset' all of that in days or weeks. It takes time and respecting the process.

This is where green flags really matter. They help you stay focused on what truly compounds over time. The behaviours you can repeat. The actions that fit your life as it is, not as you wish it were. The small, consistent choices that quietly move you forward, day after day. I'm not sure about you, but if I have the option to have more consistent energy across the week, and more on the weekend with my daughter, I am taking that any day of the week because that is the stuff that really matters.

A useful way to test this is to pay attention to how a behaviour feels. When you take a particular action, do you have more energy or less? When you skip it, what happens next?

Let me give you an example.

Case study: Self-awareness as a path to progress

Jeff, a businessman and rally car driver, was fasting most mornings when we started working together. He had heard this was a good thing, and one of his goals was weight loss. At the same time, his broader goals were to lose 3 to 5 kilograms, gain muscle, reduce body fat, come off his blood pressure medication and improve his performance in the gym.

Jeff was training with a personal trainer five mornings a week. By fasting before and after those sessions, he was not optimising

(continued)

his fuel going into training or his recovery afterwards. What he was doing had worked to a point, but as the saying goes, what got you here will not get you there.

At first, Jeff had some hesitation to change. He had built a routine, and it had delivered him results up until now. But he was willing to trust the process. Rather than changing everything at once, we agreed that on his hardest training days he would experiment with fuelling before his session and having a proper recovery breakfast within 30 to 60 minutes afterwards.

He did this consistently for two weeks. When we checked in, I asked him the same questions I asked you earlier. When you take a particular action, do you feel more energy or less? When you skip it, what happens?

The answer was immediately clear to him. On the days he fuelled and recovered properly, he had more energy in his sessions and across the rest of the day. His appetite was more stable, and even though he was eating more earlier in the day to support training and performance, it had a positive flow-on effect. His lunch and dinner were smaller, and his cravings were noticeably reduced.

On the days he fasted, his energy was less consistent, his lunch was larger and cravings were stronger later in the day.

This is what building self-awareness is all about. It helps you see what compounds for you, what is moving the needle, and brings you back to the present to assess what is working for you right now. Those green flags compound, and this is how progress not only happens, but lasts. Green flags help turn behaviours into rhythms, and rhythms into our daily operating system, showing us which areas of our life they are positively impacting.

Green flags are evidence. They are proof that something is working, even if the end goal is still a way off. This is why self-awareness sits underneath every change that lasts. It turns effort into insight, insight into action, and action into habits that actually fit your life.

This is where we stop setting ourselves up for failure, and referencing what worked for us ten years ago in different seasons of life, and we start building an operating system that supports the current version of us and our future health. That is where real, sustainable performance and wellbeing begin.

Activity

Reflect on the following questions:

- Using figure 2.1 from page 27, what signs and signals has your body been communicating to you that you have been ignoring or unsure how to interpret?
- Of the three subjective metrics (energy, appetite and performance), which one matters most to you, or speaks the most to you as your biggest opportunity to notice change? *As you make changes, tune into that metric, in particular.*
- Do you often get sick at the worst time, such as before something important or two days into the holiday you've been looking forward to?
- Do you think using a wearable device would be helpful to corroborate how you're feeling to decide when you might need to pull back to avoid getting sick?

Conclusion

Learning to listen to your body and brain is about understanding that your physiology is trying to communicate with you daily. This language is made up of signs and signals that is completely personalised to you.

When you don't understand the language, or ignore it, the signs and signals don't go away. They get louder. Pushing through can work for a period of time, until it doesn't.

When you begin to listen, the way you operate shifts. You start to recognise patterns, and you gain clarity on what supports your energy and what quietly drains it. Small, consistent decisions begin to shape how you feel, how you perform and how you recover. Self-awareness becomes practical and a genuine performance advantage.

Self-awareness allows you to adapt in busy or demanding seasons and it makes behaviour change easier as you are focused on the process, looking out for the green flags. It's important to learn to listen before you really start operating in the red.

In the next chapter, we build on this self-awareness by learning how to work with your biology rather than against it. When you do this, everything begins to feel more easeful, more sustainable and far more effective. Green flags!

Chapter Three

Finding your rhythm

Before we look at what you can upgrade, optimise or embed, we need to look at what you can leverage, which means looking at the biological rhythms that are available to you right now.

For more than 200 000 years, our ancestors lived in environments governed by light and darkness, movement and rest, feast and scarcity, and predictable daily and seasonal rhythms. Most of the dramatic changes to how we live, work and operate have occurred in just the last few hundred years, while our underlying biology has remained largely unchanged.

Our world has transformed rapidly and, with it, the way we spend our days. If you compare this to Palaeolithic times, which I have done in table 3.1 (overleaf), the contrast is significant.

Despite the huge change in environment and external cues, our biological systems responsible for keeping us alive and functioning still operate as they did thousands of years ago. They have not upgraded simply because the environment around us has.

Take for example our stress response. The fight-or-flight system evolved to deal with immediate physical threats, such as a lion or sabre-toothed tiger. It was designed to switch on quickly and switch off just as fast once the threat had passed.

Table 3.1 ***Comparison of contemporary daily habits compared with Palaeolithic humans***

	Palaeolithic times	**Today**
Light exposure	Natural light cycles aligned with sunrise and sunset	Artificial light extends the day
Food availability	Scarce and seasonal, requiring hunting and gathering	Constant availability
Movement demands	Physically varied, integrated into daily survival	Prolonged sitting and cognitively demanding work
Stress	Short, acute stress in response to immediate danger	Chronic psychological stress
Recovery and rest	Forced and unavoidable	Optional, often postponed until forced

Today, that same system is activated by constant, low-grade stressors like emails, deadlines, notifications, ongoing decision-making or the 847 emails and messages we get for Black Friday sales. This low-level activation leaves no clear opportunity to downregulate unless we intentionally live by design.

The result is a growing mismatch between how we live and the biology we operate within. This chapter is about understanding this mismatch and learning how you can live proactively and by design, and work with your biology rather than against it, to find more rhythm.

I like to start by focusing on the already existing opportunities to work with your biology before diving into your five key rhythms of nutrition, exercise, stress and recovery, sleep and connection, because leveraging what is already available to us is easier than constantly upgrading, optimising or embedding something new.

And, in my experience, these are some of the most overlooked and least understood opportunities that exist.

How did your biology evolve?

Our biology is still fundamentally the same as it was thousands of years ago when we lived as hunter-gatherers.

Back then, we moved regularly. Hunting, gathering, finding water, moving between shelter and food sources all required frequent, low-level movement. Today, we need to design our day intentionally to seek out movement, otherwise, it is very easy to spend our days sitting.

Our ancestors were exposed to natural light and darkness. There were no light switches in the caves they took shelter in. This meant their days were shaped by sunrise and sunset, which led to our biology using those light cues to regulate energy, alertness and sleep.

Back then, they experienced periods of effort when they were hunting for food or moving away from danger followed by periods of rest. Because of this, there were times that required focus, exertion and intensity, and times that allowed for recovery and downshifting.

As a result, our nervous systems evolved to handle short bursts of stress. Stress would rise quickly in response to a threat, resolve and then settle. What we were never designed for is constant stimulation, constant decision-making and constant low-grade stress, like the pings, dings and demands we are exposed to today.

The challenge is that, while the world around us has changed dramatically, these biological systems have not. When we ignore this, stress and strain escalate under the surface due to the misalignment. As a result, your energy may become unpredictable, your focus harder to sustain, and you're left feeling tired but wired as a result of always being on and never being fully rested.

This is why finding your rhythm matters.

One of the biggest problems I see is people operating in an unsustainable way. Often there is a quiet narrative that they are the exception to the rule. I used to believe this myself. But after more than 15 years working with thousands of high performers, one thing is clear: no matter how exceptional you are, you are not invincible.

Sure, for a period, you can operate in the red and survive off long days fuelled by caffeine, cortisol and adrenaline. Even with minimal sleep and constant pressure, you can still meet deadlines and deliver results. But this pace always comes at a cost. That cost may show up quickly as burnout or breakdown, or much later as long-term health consequences.

I know what you might be thinking: *My workload has never been higher. I am at capacity. It requires more of me and that's just the reality.* But there is a critical difference between working harder and working smarter.

Working with your biology is the smarter option. It allows you to have more energy, greater focus and higher productivity, while still preserving energy for what matters most: your health, relationships and your life outside of work.

Learning to go with your natural flow

When you work with your biology, things feel easier and more effortless relative to how they feel now. I often describe it like swimming with the current. You move faster with less effort and arrive with more energy left in the tank. That is working smarter.

When you work against your biology, it feels like swimming against the current. Everything takes more effort than it should, not to mention it takes longer to get where you're going and you arrive more exhausted. You still get to where you're going, but it costs you more time, more effort and more energy.

So, which would you prefer?

This chapter is about learning to swim with the current of life by leveraging your biology. Central to this are three biological rhythms that quietly shape how you feel and perform every day. You may have heard of one or more of them. But I suspect, like most people I have worked with or supported, it is unlikely you are proactively and intentionally designing your days around them.

The three biological rhythms we are going to explore are your:

1. circadian rhythm
2. sleep chronotype
3. ultradian rhythm.

Your circadian rhythm

Have you ever been camping or been to a health retreat and noticed that you go to bed much earlier than normal? If you have, this is likely the closest you've come to true circadian alignment.

Regardless of whether you're more of a health retreat person or a camping one, the outcome is often the same. Artificial light is removed, technology is limited and your days and activities naturally follow the sun rising and setting.

I remember arriving at a health retreat where we were told to expect to feel exhausted after dinner and that we'd all go to bed earlier than usual. I was in the Gold Coast hinterland, with no phones due to poor reception, no laptops and no televisions in the room. By 7.30 pm, when the sun had set and it was dark, everyone was ready for sleep. Even for someone who is normally in bed by 9 pm, this was a new experience.

I remember how much this resonated with me and how it has stayed with me as a powerful reminder of how effective it is to work with your biology, and how strongly your circadian rhythm responds when the environment supports it.

Your circadian rhythm is your internal 24-hour clock. It governs your sleep-wake cycle, but it also influences a wide range of hormonal, metabolic and cognitive processes across the day, including energy levels, alertness, appetite regulation, focus and recovery.

As Matthew Walker explains in his book *Why We Sleep*,[11] sleep and wakefulness are regulated by two key biological forces:

1. sleep pressure, driven by a chemical called adenosine
2. circadian rhythm, which acts as your internal timing system.

In simple terms, sleep pressure is your body's built-up need for sleep that increases the longer you've been awake. Your circadian rhythm provides the signal for when your brain and body should be awake and alert, and the cascade of physiological processes that happen because of that.

The biggest external cue for your circadian rhythm is light.

Light entering your eyes sends information directly to the brain, which determines what time of day it is, and which physiological processes should be prioritised. When light is present, the message is be awake, alert and productive. When light fades, the signal shifts toward recovery and rest. Historically, the sun rising and setting were the main cues we had.

One of the simplest and highest-return behaviours for supporting your circadian rhythm is exposure to natural light early in the day, signalling that it is time to get up and get going with your day. Similarly, light exposure as the sun begins to set signals that its getting closer to bed time.

Getting ten to 15 minutes of daylight into your eyes as soon as possible after waking is one of the most effective ways to support energy and cognitive output across the day. This means, where possible, outdoor light, and ideally, not through a window, sunglasses or artificial light, just natural daylight exposure. We're lucky in Australia, as throughout the year, even in our winter months, there is still approximately nine to 11 hours a day of light exposure.

This single input of morning light triggers a cascade of physiological responses, including support for:

- a healthy rise in cortisol (the hormone that helps the body wake, engage and perform)
- increased release of serotonin (your feel-good hormone responsible for supporting mood, motivation and focus)
- suppression of residual melatonin (your sleepy hormone responsible for helping you get to sleep).

Cortisol often gets a bad reputation, but in the morning, it plays an essential role in helping you feel awake, focused and ready to engage with the day. When cortisol rises at the right time, energy feels more stable and alertness more sustained. The issue is when our cortisol rhythm is out of alignment and remains elevated later in the day, disrupting sleep, recovery and emotional regulation.

Dr Andrew Huberman talks about the importance of getting your cortisol rhythm right on his podcast *Huberman Lab*. Dr Huberman states you want 'to make sure your highest levels of cortisol [are] in the morning upon waking and in the first few hours of the morning, which will help improve your energy, your focus and your learning across the day.'[12]

Morning light also supports serotonin activity across the day. That same serotonin acts as a precursor to melatonin, the hormone that helps prepare the body for sleep. Roughly 14 to 16 hours after morning light exposure, the serotonin produced earlier drives the natural release of melatonin in the evening, provided light exposure is adjusted as the day winds down.

The outcome of this morning light exposure is simple but powerful: better energy during the day and better sleep readiness at night. All from a behaviour that takes minutes.

One of the challenges we face today is the constant exposure to artificial light. Screens, overhead lighting and late-night device use blur the signals our brain relies on to keep time and regulate our circadian rhythm. Where our ancestors only had access to sunlight and firelight, we now live in environments that tell the brain it is daytime well into the evening.

The result is disruption to our physiology. Melatonin release is delayed, downshifting becomes harder and, at a biological level, we struggle to recognise when it is time to rest. We will explore this in more detail in Chapter 7 when we discuss your sleep rhythm.

If you travel regularly for work or pleasure, your circadian rhythm is disrupted and this contributes to jet lag. Light is the strongest signal your brain uses to reset its internal clock. Used intentionally, light exposure is one of the most effective tools for reducing how long you are jet lagged for and restoring your circadian rhythm.

Aligning more with the natural rise and fall of daylight is about anchoring your day to a biological signal your brain is already primed to look for. Working with your circadian rhythm is one of the highest-return upgrades you can make. It improves performance during the day and recovery at night. Green flags!

Tip: Your circadian rhythm essentials

- Morning: Aim for ten to 15 minutes of sunlight on your eyes soon after waking.
- Daytime: Get natural light in the earlier afternoon and avoid prolonged bright light late in the day.
- Evening: Dim lights and reduce screen time 60 to 90 minutes before bed.

Your sleep chronotype

While your circadian rhythm largely governs the day, your sleep chronotype is a more personal biological rhythm. It determines what time of day you are naturally most alert and focused, and your ideal wake time and bedtime.

Your chronotype reflects your body's natural timing for alertness and sleep. It explains why some people feel sharp early, others peak later and many sit somewhere in between.

Research shows that while most people experience predictable rises and falls in energy and focus across the day, the timing of those peaks is not universal. We all move through natural cycles of alertness and fatigue, but where those crests and slumps occur depends on your chronotype.[13]

Understanding your chronotype, and aligning when you wake, when you go to sleep and when you do your most cognitively demanding work, is the definition of working smarter, not harder, and another way you can work with your biology.

Some people are biologically wired to feel alert earlier in the day, while others naturally peak later. While your chronotype can shift slightly across different stages of life, deliberately retraining it is difficult and rarely sustainable as there is a strong genetic component.

Most of us fall into one of four chronotype profiles, as described by psychologist Michael Breus (also known as the Sleep Doctor)[14]:

- Lions: Morning types. Early to bed, early to rise. Peak productivity in the morning.
- Bears: Align with the sun, most productive midday between 10 am and 2 pm.
- Wolves: Evening types. Later to rise, later to sleep. Peak productivity after lunch.
- Dolphins: Rare; often light sleepers who struggle with insomnia. Those with less consistent energy rhythms.

Each profile has different windows for wake time, most productive time and sleep time, which has been summarised in table 3.2 (adapted from Michael Breus's work).

Table 3.2 *Sleep chronotypes*

	Lions (15–20%)	**Bears (55%)**	**Wolves (15–20%)**	**Dolphins (10%)**
Wake up	<6 am	7 am	7.30 am	6.30 am
Most productive	8 am–2 pm	10 am–2 pm	1 pm–5 pm	10 am–2 pm
Bedtime	<10 pm	11 pm	12 am	11.30 pm

Note: Percentages indicate approximate proportion of the population that falls into each category.

Looking at the chronotypes, I am sure you intuitively have a pretty good sense of which chronotype you are, and if you aren't typically a morning person or an evening person, you most likely sit in the middle.

Knowing your chronotype presents you with an opportunity to align your most important work with your most productive window, which can help you place the right work in the right hours, and work more efficiently.

For me, as a lion chronotype, I always try and do my 'deep' project work in the morning, because that is my most productive window.

These chronotypes are also why the idea of one-size-fits-all productivity protocols that mandate practices such as 'eat the frog first' or subscribing to the 5 AM Club[15] are not ideal. Biologically, these approaches simply do not work for everyone.

Sure, they may work well for around 15 to 20 per cent of the population who are natural morning types, such as lions. But for other chronotypes, forcing early wake times or doing the most demanding work first thing in the morning is not working smarter. It is working against their biology and it can have them feeling like they are swimming against the current.

If an opportunity exists for you to align some of your tasks or part of your day with your chronotype, give it a try. Tune in to those subjective metrics and see how you feel. My bet is you will find it feels more like you are in alignment and swimming with the current, rather than against it.

Tip: Your sleep chronotype essentials

- Notice when you naturally wake, feel most alert and like to go to sleep — that's likely your sleep chronotype.
- Wherever possible, schedule your most important or demanding tasks into those peak focus windows.
- Protect your sleep by keeping a consistent sleep-wake window that suits your chronotype rather than forcing an idealised schedule.

Your ultradian rhythm

What does your current work calendar look like?

Let me take a guess. Back-to-back meetings, some in-person, most on Zoom. One call finishes and the next begins. In between, there might be a quick coffee, a scroll through social media or a rush to clear emails before the next meeting starts. Lunch isn't at a set time and is often eaten at your desk or sometimes skipped altogether.

The front half of your day feels pretty good. You're focused. You're moving quickly, responding, making decisions and staying on top of things. Then, almost without warning, something shifts. Focus becomes harder to hold, thinking feels fuzzy, you reread the same email multiple times. Your energy and cognitive capacity dip even though your day is far from over. You think, I need that extra coffee today, and your eye is drawn to the sweet treat on the counter. Carbs and caffeine should do the trick!

If you feel seen, I've got you! What is happening under the surface is that you are relying on heightened arousal to maintain output. Stress hormones and stimulants can keep you going for a period of time, but without moments to downregulate, which you can think of as recovery pauses, that effort is difficult to sustain and requires a lot of push effort and external stimulants, which is not sustainable.

This is the result of working in a way that ignores your third biological rhythm: your ultradian rhythm.

This rhythm operates beneath the surface of the day. Your energy does not run in a straight line. It moves in waves and micro cycles. Roughly every 90 minutes, you move through periods of higher performance followed by a natural dip lasting around 20 minutes, before the cycle begins again. You can see what this looks like in figure 3.1.

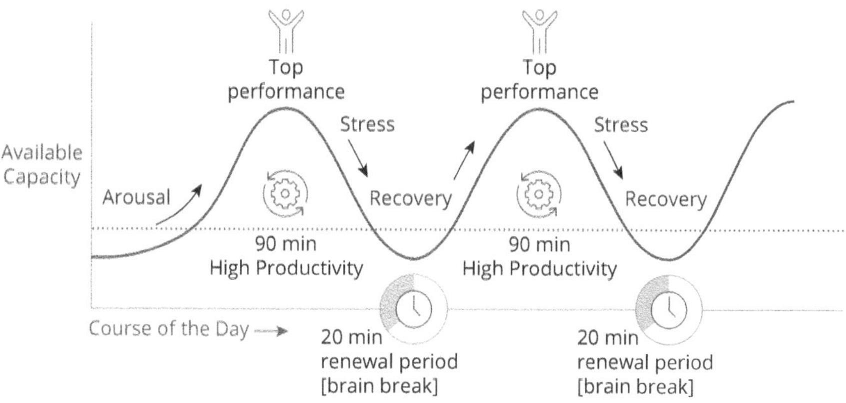

Figure 3.1 *Ultradian rhythms*

If I am honest, leveraging this biological rhythm is the strategy I am using to write this book. I aim to structure my workdays this way — and most days, I do. Some days I don't, and that's okay (I am human, after all). How I like to leverage this rhythm is by working with a timer. I set it for 90 minutes of focused writing in my performance pulse, then I deliberately stop for a recovery pause. During that time, I might go for a walk, go to the gym or sauna, have a meal or snack or a cup of tea or listen to a meditation track. I like to mix it up.

Working this way allows me to focus deeply, get into the zone and then reset before starting again. This is how, biologically, we are designed to operate at our best, and when we know this, coupled with our sleep chronotype, we can design our workflow around it. I can't wait for you to try it!

While it's common to operate in a linear way, with back-to-back stimulation in the form of screens, meetings, caffeine hits and emails, biologically, we are much better suited to operating in pulses: a performance pulse followed by a recovery pulse. This is another way you can start to work smarter, not harder, and swim with the current!

The problem is that most of us ignore the dip and push straight through it with more stimulation. That might look like more screen time, scrolling on social media, more caffeine, a quick check of the inbox while waiting for lunch. Over time, this pattern leads to cognitive fatigue, poorer decision-making and the familiar feeling of being constantly busy, flat and depleted.

Working with your ultradian rhythm means allowing brief moments to downshift during those dips. Even short pauses, without additional stimulation, can help reset the system enough to perform well again.

Knowing when to pause allows you to perform at a high level for longer. Even Formula 1 cars need pit stops, ideally proactive and strategic ones, rather than reactive stops caused by technical issues. Humans are no different.

Tip: Your ultradian rhythm essentials

- Try working in pulses across your day made up of a performance pulse, followed by a recovery pulse.

- You can choose the exact length and rhythm based on what works for your day, but aiming for about 90 minutes of focused work followed by a short recovery pulse is a great place to aim for.

At this point, the goal is not to change everything you do, it is simply to understand this rhythm and start noticing how it shows up in your own day. You simply need to notice when the dip arrives, respect it and take an intentional pause. On page 141, we will look at how to schedule these moments into your day. A key part of building your operating system is not relying on willpower or hoping the day allows for a break, but creating a proactive system that supports you by design.

In the sections that follow, we will explore how to build recovery into your day in a way that fits your life, whether you have one minute, three minutes, or ten to 20. The key is not the duration, it is that recovery is present, intentional and proactive.

I am yet to meet someone who regrets creating more space to recover during the day! Most people find it surprisingly enjoyable and quickly notice clearer thinking, steadier energy and a greater sense of control over how they move through their day.

Activity

Let's do a biological rhythm audit to see what opportunities exist for you to work more in alignment with your biology.

- Do I get ten to 15 minutes of sunlight on my eyes within 30 to 60 minutes of waking (or as early as possible once the sun rises)?

(continued)

- Do I dim the lights and reduce exposure to screens 60 to 90 minutes before going to bed?
- Am I a lion, bear, wolf or dolphin chronotype?
- Based on the chronotype I innately know I am, is there an opportunity to work smarter rather than harder?
- Do I currently work in pulses (performance pulse, followed by a recovery pulse) or a flat-line linear approach?
- If I were to start working in pulses, what cadence do I think would work for me for my performance pulse and my recovery pulse (e.g., 90-minute performance pulse, five to ten-minute recovery pulse).

Conclusion

Our bodies already know how to regulate energy, focus and recovery. They have been doing so for thousands of years, largely unchanged. What has changed is the environment we live in.

Learning how to work with key internal biological rhythms helps you work smarter, rather than harder.

Working with your circadian rhythm brings structure to your day. Energy and effort are better supported earlier, while the evening naturally becomes a time for downshifting and recovery, with light being the strongest external cue we have.

When you take your sleep chronotype into account and align when you wake, sleep and tackle your highest priority work with your most productive windows, effort decreases and output improves.

When you look to structure your day with performance pulses followed by recovery pulses, this allows you to sustain energy, output and focus while you are 'on' and then allows for downshifts and restoration during your intentional stimulant-free time. This structure of pulses sustains energy and capacity across your day and week.

Now that you understand these three biological rhythms that already exist and how they help influence energy, focus and recovery, we can turn our attention to the five key rhythms that make up your operating system: nutrition, exercise, stress and recovery, sleep and connection.

Part 2

The 5 rhythms of your operating system

Chapter Four

Nutrition — Fuelling wellbeing and performance

Imagine if there was something you already did every single day, multiple times per day, that directly impacted your energy, mood, focus, performance and wellbeing that also happened to be one of the biggest levers when it comes to your health — and it's something you enjoy!

Well, there is, and that thing is your nutrition.

Eating is one of the few behaviours you do every single day, multiple times per day, yet in my experience, it is often very misunderstood by people.

Case study: Setting your foundation

Take Marnie, a managing director and mother of two, who came to me because she felt like she was running on empty and was struggling to stay focused through her work day. This was

(continued)

frustrating because she exercised regularly, she cooked most meals and ate 'pretty well'. She couldn't work out why she'd gained a few kilograms and just felt flat.

When she completed her life audit template for the week (a process I use with my coaching clients), what stood out was not *what* she was eating, it was how inconsistently she was eating day to day, and in particular, how her morning started. There were about four different versions. Some mornings she would have breakfast at home at 7 am, other days in the office about 9 am. Some days it might only be scraps off her kids' plates as she was about to leave for school drop-off, and there were the occasional mornings of nothing. Lunchtime varied depending on how hungry she was and what meetings she had, and whether she was working from home or in the office.

When we started to uncover how different her nutrition inputs were each day, in particular in the morning, it started to click why her energy, appetite and cravings were inconsistent.

Over three months, Marnie upgraded various aspects of her nutrition rhythm, but the most significant one for her was stabilising and standardising what she did at breakfast. She needed a few options that all gave her what she needed but worked for the different mornings and days she had — when she worked from home or the office, when she dropped the kids to school, when she trained and when she didn't. When she got this locked in, the entire trajectory of her day shifted for the better.

This is where a lot of people go wrong with their nutrition. They assume nutrition is only about what you eat. Don't get me wrong, the quality of what you eat matters, but the rhythm and the consistency of how you eat, especially when it comes to your energy, is equally, if not more, important.

This is why nutrition has such a powerful impact on how you feel day to day, and how it ripples into every aspect of wellbeing and performance. The best part is that nutrition is about so much more than food. It is social connection, it creates experience and memories, and it's enjoyable. And none of that needs to change.

This chapter is about understanding how to leverage nutrition to support better energy, sharper focus, enhanced mood and improved performance in every aspect of life.

When you use nutrition as a consistent foundation and starting point for your day, both with what you eat and the timing, it consistently kick starts your morning. The rhythm with which you then eat across the day largely determines how consistent your energy levels are, which largely impacts your focus.

It was my own personal experience that first taught me how powerful nutrition is when it comes to your health and performance. So much so, that it set me on the trajectory of my entire professional career.

Back when I was swimming at a national level in primary and high school, I started seeing a sports dietitian. The combination of heavy training loads and puberty left me with low iron, low energy, constant fatigue and frequent sickness. My parents were doing their best to support me, but none of us really knew what I needed. It's hard to approximate what is needed to fuel four hours in a pool a day on top of puberty!

That was the first time I experienced a clear shift from feeling exhausted, flat and low on energy to feeling fuelled, energised and focused purely through adjusting my nutrition. It showed me, very early on, just how powerful nutrition can be when it comes to your health, your performance and your energy.

There was another point in time that I ended up in hospital overnight on a drip because I was dehydrated, so despite spending my entire career helping thousands of people improve their nutrition, I also know what it feels like to get it completely wrong.

This chapter has been designed to provide you with a road map to leverage nutrition to give you more energy and to improve your overall health and performance. I encourage you to read through this chapter in order, identify your first opportunity to make an improvement, and start there.

Consistency before anything else

As we've discussed, your body operates best with predictable patterns. Take for instance how you eat. Consistent timing with your meals and snacks supports steadier blood glucose levels, more reliable appetite cues and more stable energy across the day.

For that reason, before you change what you are eating, you can improve your energy and wellbeing simply by changing *how* you eat.

When I talk about consistency, there are a few key inputs that you would benefit from standardising. The first is the time you start eating each day. For most people, their first meal of the day is breakfast. This is one of the most common areas of inconsistency I see in practice, and the flow-on effect of this inconsistency at the start of the day shows up as greater disruptions to energy or appetite in the afternoon or evening like it did with Marnie.

Marnie is not alone. This is one of the most common patterns I see and hear today, and hybrid work has only made it more challenging.

At least when we had to be at the same location (the office) at the same time, it standardised our days, which helped stabilise our behaviours. While flexible work has been a gift in so many ways, the one area it has caused chaos for a lot of people is in their behaviours and rhythms.

An equation that is important for you to understand is this: you cannot expect consistent outputs, like energy, if the inputs going into the equation, like your eating behaviours, are inconsistent.

In Marnie's example, having various breakfasts at varying times was resulting in low and inconsistent energy levels. Completely different inputs led to inconsistent and draining energy levels. If you want consistent energy, you need more consistent inputs.

Think about the key consistent nutrition inputs for you to focus on, such as the:

- time of the day you start eating
- time of the day you stop eating
- number of meals and snacks you have across the day
- gaps (time/hours) between each of those meals and snacks.

To be clear, this is not about being a robot or eating the exact same foods at the exact same time every day. That is rigidity and is not setting you up with the tools for success. The way you want to think about these consistent behaviours is similar to guardrails.

The time you start and stop eating does not need to be exact, but aim for within a 30- to 60-minute window. This should also guide the timing between your meals and snacks. As a guide to get you started, around four hours is a good gap for most people, but that range might go down to three hours or up to five hours. This creates a more consistent rhythm of meals and snacks across the day, which will drive more consistent energy and appetite.

When you do this, don't just focus on weekdays. The weekends can be the trickiest times for people without them even realising it. Again, this is not about needing to apply the exact same strategy to the weekend, but if your weekend is unpredictable and there is zero consistency with what you eat and when, having an understanding of that to start is important, and thinking about how you can apply the same principles in a way that works is helpful.

Reflection

Reflect on these questions and answer them for your weekdays and weekends.

- What time do you start eating on the different days across the week?
- What time do you stop eating on the different days across the week?
- If you were to standardise these times between a 30- to 60-minute window, what would that look like?
- On days I feel my best, how many meals and snacks does that include?

All the Elements

Once the foundation of consistency with how you eat is in place, the next question becomes *what should I eat?*

Is it just me or do recommendations around this seem to be changing constantly? One day carbohydrates are the problem, the next day it's fat. Then it is timing, fasting, supplements. It's no wonder that most of us end up getting confused and overwhelmed and then just keep doing what we were doing.

After working with over 1000 elite athletes, executives, leaders and Special Forces operators, I realised something important: people do not need more nutrition information. They need a simple structure that removes guesswork that they can apply in real time, regardless of where they are and what they are doing.

That led to me to develop All the Elements.

All the Elements is a practical framework for building meals and snacks that consistently supports energy, performance, recovery today, as well as for your long-term health. It works whether you are fuelling for elite sport, a demanding leadership role or simply trying to feel better in your day-to-day life.

While most diets or trends focus on some form of restriction, All the Elements focuses on inclusion and understanding why each food type is important.

Instead of asking what you should cut out, All the Elements asks: *What do I need to include?* When meals are built with All the Elements consistently, you really start to understand how food works with you to support your energy, focus, performance and long-term wellbeing—not to mention it is satisfying, tasty and simple.

With All the Elements:

- energy becomes more stable
- appetite (and cravings) are easier to manage
- focus improves
- decision-making becomes less reactive as you have a framework.

Green flags!

Here's the thing, the food you eat at a meal or as a snack does not just affect you the moment you eat it, or just after. It impacts how you feel hours later, even the next day. For example, what you do (or don't eat) in the morning will show up in the afternoon or early evening. Remember those cravings we discussed in Chapter 2, and how I don't believe in them? This is part of that equation.

This is the flow-on effect. The decisions you make at breakfast or in the morning show up at lunchtime or mid-afternoon. Lunch shows up at 3 pm or before dinner. Dinner shows up in your sleep, or all of it shows up the next day.

When you have a consistent rhythm with what you eat, and then you layer in the All the Elements framework to each meal and snack, food starts to become your consistent energy booster and appetite satisfier. The shift is remarkable, and it also happens very quickly—as in the same day!

So, what are these elements I speak about?

The four elements

Every meal, and most snacks, should contain four key elements. For the time being, we'll identify what they are and why they are important. Once this becomes second nature, there are some nuances to when these elements and the ratios adjust, which I touch on later in this chapter.

But for the stage we are at, let's look at what they are and which foods sit in each element.

Protein

Protein is the foundation. It plays a central role in building and maintaining muscle, supporting physical recovery, stabilising blood sugar, regulating appetite, and sustaining focus and energy across the day.

It is also the element most people under-prioritise early in the day, and as a consequence, overload on it at night. With your protein intake, you want to spread it out evenly across the day. I will dive more into the details of this in the protein pulsing section on page 80, but for the purpose of this section, that's what you need to know.

When your protein intake is optimised, meaning you have a consistent amount at each meal and snack, you notice the difference quickly. Nearly instantly! Across the day you will have more stable energy, and if there is a particular time of day you get really hungry or have cravings, those will reduce, or maybe even disappear, as protein helps you to be more satiated.

High-quality protein foods include meat, poultry, seafood, dairy products, soy-based products, lentils, legumes, and also good-quality protein powders.

Carbohydrates

Carbohydrates are often misunderstood. They are the primary fuel source for the brain and working muscles. While the brain accounts for only around 2 per cent of body weight, it uses approximately 20 per cent of the body's energy. It is an energy-hungry organ!

Carbohydrates also play a critical role in blood glucose regulation. When high-quality, high-fibre carbohydrates are consumed in more consistent amounts across the day, and matched to our outputs, they help stabilise energy, mood and focus. When poorly timed or unbalanced, they can drive energy crashes and cravings.

Wholegrain, high-fibre carbohydrates are especially important, not only for energy regulation but also for gut health, which we will explore later in this chapter.

High-fibre carbohydrate foods you want to prioritise include wholegrains, legumes, lentils, fruit and vegetables.

Colours

Colours is my way of talking about fruits and vegetables. It's important to understand that the different colours of fruits and vegetables reflect different micronutrients. For example, purple-coloured fruits and vegetables are rich in anthocyanins, a powerful antioxidant linked with recovery and anti-inflammatory properties, whereas those that are orange and yellow are rich in beta carotene (Vitamin A).

The colours in fruits and vegetables provide a range of important anti-inflammatory compounds for our body, including vitamins, minerals, antioxidants, polyphenols and bioactive compounds that support immunity, cellular health, gut diversity and long-term vitality.

These foods are also packed with various types of fibres that fill us up for longer. The different types of fibre are also the types of food our good gut bugs like to feast on, which we will cover in more detail on page 83.

While 'eat more colour' sounds simple, what this is communicating is a much more complex and important message for our overall health, performance and energy.

> ***Tip: All the colours***
>
> If a meal or snack is brown and white, it is not complete. Think about ways to add colour: a side salad, some berries on top, a handful of spinach. Anything colourful is a huge gain in boosting the nutrient diversity of your meal or snack.

Healthy fats

Healthy fats are often neglected or avoided unnecessarily. They are essential for absorbing fat-soluble vitamins (A, E, D and K), supporting hormone health, reducing inflammation and improving satiety. They also make food enjoyable, which is an important part of you being consistent with what you eat. You need to enjoy it!

When fats are included appropriately, meals are more satisfying, appetite is more stable and energy regulation improves. Green flags!

Healthy fats include our poly- and monounsaturated fats like extra virgin olive oil, avocado, nuts and seeds, and oily fish.

Figure 4.1 shows the four elements, the types of foods in each category and the key role each element plays.

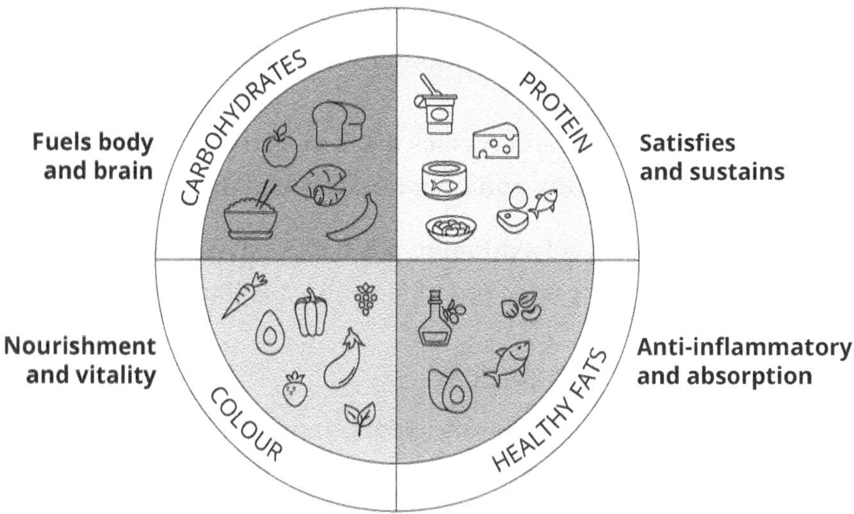

Figure 4.1 *All the Elements*

If you can apply this framework to each meal and most snacks, you will start to feel the difference it makes to your energy, appetite and performance (your subjective metrics) very quickly.

All the Elements is a tool to help simplify what you eat to support your health, performance and longevity without complexity like having to track your meals. Another practical upgrade that aligns closely with this approach is food sequencing.

Food sequencing

This is another example of how you don't even have to change what you are eating, just how you eat, and you can get a win when it comes to your energy levels.

Starting your meal with the protein and vegetables (colours), and then eating the carbohydrate component last has a range of benefits, including:

- slowing digestion and blunting the post-meal blood glucose response
- reducing spikes and crashes that can lead to afternoon fatigue, irritability and poor decision-making.[16]

This means you can get a different physiological response by eating the same meal in a specific order! How great is that?

To snack or not to snack?

In my opinion, snacks are one of the most misunderstood and underutilised areas of nutrition. When done well, a strategic and satisfying snack plays an important role in supporting energy across the day, particularly in the afternoon.

The reason I say that is, it's common for the gap between breakfast and lunch to usually be much shorter than the gap between lunch and dinner. For example, breakfast might be 8 am and lunch at 12 pm, around four hours apart. But lunch to dinner might be six or seven hours.

In my experience, many people underestimate that second gap. They either have nothing at all, or they rely on something small and insufficient to carry them through. A coffee, a couple of biscuits, or a light snack might take the edge off briefly, but none of these provide enough protein or fibre to stabilise your blood sugar levels, your appetite or your focus for several hours.

This approach often creates a predictable 'flow-on effect'. You arrive at dinner overly hungry, eat a larger portion than you intended, and are more likely to reach for something sweet or savoury before or after your meal.

A better option from a rhythm perspective would be to have an intentional, proactive afternoon snack, around 3 pm or 4 pm. One that fuels you, satisfies you, supports stable energy and focus through the afternoon—and also has you arriving at dinner ready to eat, but not starving. Green flags!

The research is clear that it is not snacking itself that matters, but the timing and quality. Higher-quality snacks consumed earlier in the day are associated with healthier lipid and insulin responses, while late-evening snacking is linked with poorer glycaemic control.[17]

A high-quality snack does not need to be complicated. I encourage you to aim for three or four key elements: protein, colours, and either high-fibre carbohydrates or healthy fats. Bonus points if you can include all four. Foods like fruit, yoghurt, nuts, seeds and whole grains support better nutrient distribution across the day and are associated with improved cardiometabolic markers when used intentionally.

When your body can anticipate what is coming, it does not need to react to energy dips, long meeting blocks or diary gaps. That predictability alone goes a long way toward stabilising appetite and blood glucose. And when those are stable, energy tends to follow, before you even change a single food choice.

Figure 4.2 is an example of someone who skips breakfast, has a small breakfast or is experimenting with intermittent fasting. Mid-morning they might have a coffee and a piece of fruit. As the day goes on their meals become progressively larger, as shown by the size of the bar charts.

Not only are their meals uneven in size, and trending upwards across the day, but their blood glucose levels, appetite and cravings follow the same pattern. Energy dips earlier, hunger builds more aggressively and cravings intensify later in the day.

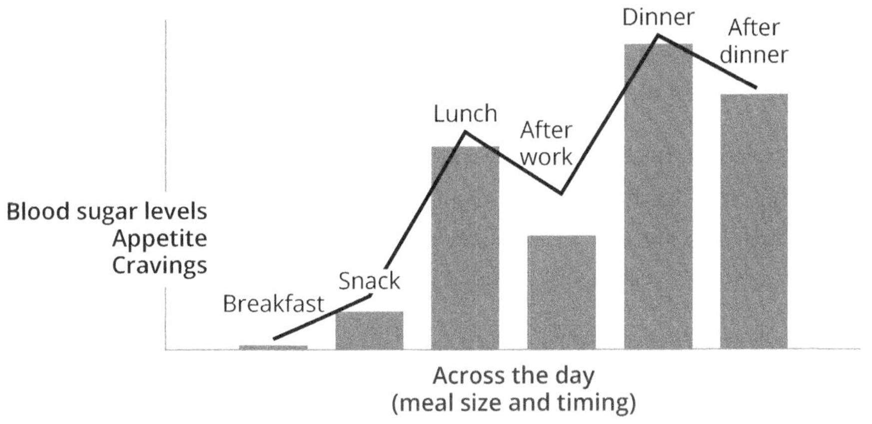

Figure 4.2 *Inconsistent food intake in a day*

When meals are more evenly distributed across the day (see figure 4.3), the benefits are significant. Eating consistently sized meals across the day creates a more stable blood glucose response, supports steadier appetite and reduces the intensity of cravings later in the day (if you experience them).

If your dinner is currently much larger than your breakfast and lunch, the goal is to gradually bring them closer in size. This does not mean halving your dinner and moving it to breakfast. It means increasing what you eat at the start of your day.

This can be uncomfortable or difficult at first, particularly if you are not used to eating earlier. But when you persist, your body adapts. Your appetite becomes more regulated, and the increased hunger that was showing up later afternoon or in the evening begins to even out.

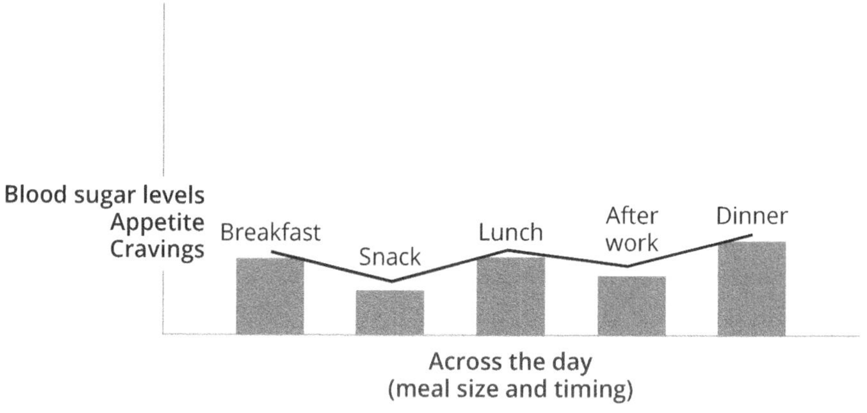

Figure 4.3 *Consistent (ideal) food intake in a day*

If you have no rhythm, no consistency with what you eat and when, and the gaps between meals and snacks is varied, you can't expect to have consistent energy levels.

Diet quality matters

Regardless of when you eat or how you eat, *what* you eat (aka diet quality) matters! Yes, this is about eating wholefoods, but it is also about removing a category of foods as much as possible—ultra-processed foods.

The NOVA classification system (see figure 4.4) groups foods based on the degree of processing. The category of greatest concern is Group 4: ultra-processed foods. These are products typically characterised by long ingredient lists, industrial additives, emulsifiers and flavourings, with little resemblance to whole food in its original form.[18]

In Australia, a significant proportion of our daily energy intake now comes from ultra-processed foods, with even higher intakes seen in younger adults and more disadvantaged groups. In many Western countries, ultra-processed foods account for around half or more of the total daily energy intake.[19]

Large-scale reviews have consistently shown that higher consumption of ultra-processed foods are associated with increased risk across a wide range of health outcomes, including cardiometabolic disease, mental health conditions and all-cause mortality.[20] When relied on too heavily, they displace foods that provide fibre, micronutrients and bioactive compounds that support gut health, metabolic resilience and long-term wellbeing.

As you read this, your mind probably goes to the more obvious ultra-processed foods: the chips, biscuits, chocolate and fried foods. But there are also less-obvious options like protein bars and ready-to-drink protein shakes. Keeping this in mind becomes particularly relevant as we move into the importance of pulsing your protein, but that does not mean any type of food or protein. Quality matters!

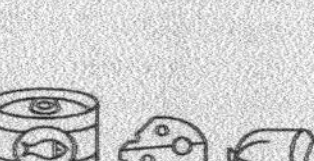
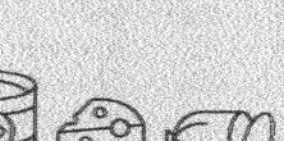
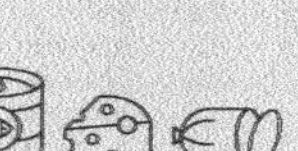
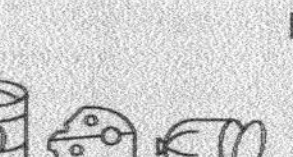
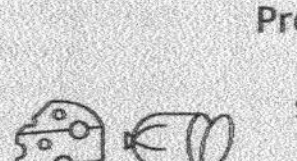
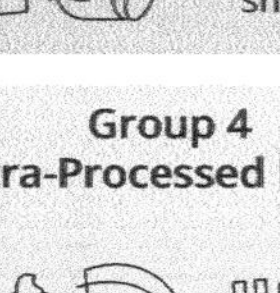
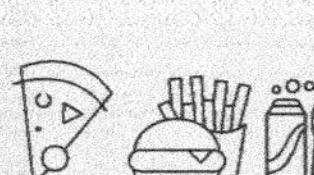
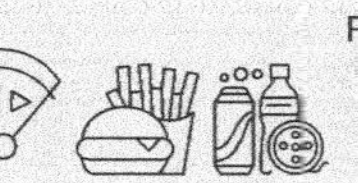

Figure 4.4 *The NOVA classification system*

Protein pulsing

Protein really deserves its own section, not because it is fashionable or on trend, but because of the key role it plays in energy, recovery and long-term health.

Protein-rich foods help regulate appetite and blood glucose, two of the biggest drivers of energy consistency across the day. When protein intake is inadequate or poorly distributed, energy becomes inconsistent. When it is consistent, your energy and appetite are much more consistent too.

This is where the concept of *protein pulsing* comes in. Protein pulsing refers to deliberately spreading your protein intake across the day, rather than consuming the majority of it in one or two sittings, typically at lunch and dinner. Research consistently shows that distributing protein more evenly supports muscle protein synthesis (your ability to grow and maintain muscle mass), improves appetite regulation, stabilises blood glucose and enhances recovery.[21] Green flags!

As a general guide, aim for between 20 and 40 grams of protein per meal or snack. For my people who want to be more specific, between 0.3 and 0.4 grams per kilogram of body weight per eating occasion. The total amount of protein to aim for per day is between 1.2 and 2.0 grams per kilogram of body weight.

For general health and wellbeing, you would aim to consume towards the lower end of those measurements; if you are lifting heavy weights, transitioning through perimenopause or menopause, ageing or using a GLP-1, you should be consuming at the higher end. Understanding good-quality foods that are rich in protein is important and something I believe everyone should upskill in.[22]

There are three reasons, in particular, why protein matters.

1. Protein plays a central role in maintaining muscle mass. Muscle is critical for metabolic health, resilience and longevity, particularly as we age. The loss of muscle mass is not linear, especially for women; periods such as perimenopause and menopause represent a time of accelerated change, making adequate protein intake, coupled with weights training (which we will touch on in Chapter 5), even more important.[23]
2. Protein supports recovery. It underpins tissue repair, adaptation to training and the ability to tolerate physical and cognitive load over time.
3. The most overlooked reason is the impact protein distribution has on energy and appetite. Protein is the most satiating macronutrient. When it is consumed consistently across the day, blood glucose is more stable, cravings are reduced and energy crashes are far less common. This means you arrive at meals hungry, but not ravenous.[24]

Of all the protein pulses across the day, your first one matters the most. A protein-rich breakfast or first meal has repeatedly been shown to support steadier energy, improved appetite control and better focus across the day.[25] Yet, in practice, it is common for protein to be under-consumed or missed due to poor planning, not liking or being good at breakfast, or fasting.

With protein, the goal is simple, at least in theory. Aim for four to five consistent pulses of protein across the day. When protein is distributed more evenly, energy steadies, appetite becomes easier to manage, focus improves and recovery is supported.

Tip: Nutrition training mindset

If increasing protein at breakfast feels challenging, think of it as nutrition training. Just like returning to the gym after time off, it takes practice, consistency and progressive exposure. You want to think about any new eating habit or upgrade to how you eat the same. It might be hard or challenging at first, but over time you adapt, it becomes easier and then eventually a habit!

A word on fasting

There is a lot that could be said here about fasting but I want to keep it short and sweet. My position on intermittent fasting is simple: it is an advanced tool for an advanced user.

Intermittent fasting is an umbrella term that includes a range of approaches, many of which involve fasting windows and more compressed eating periods. In practice, this often looks like skipping or delaying the first meal until late morning or lunch, then finishing early in the evening.

The reason I am cautious with fasting, is because it can make it harder to hit key behaviours with your nutrition rhythm that matter most for health, body composition and performance: adequate total protein, evenly distributed protein pulses across the day and sufficient fibre.

This matters because suboptimal total protein and fewer, larger protein boluses may reduce the number of anabolic 'hits' for muscle, which, over time, can compromise gaining and retaining muscle mass.[26]

In some instances, it can undermine the goals you're chasing, like it did with Jeff, who you met in Chapter 2. I have also seen it repeatedly with elite athletes who dabble with fasting on their days off to manage overall intake and body composition, including AFL player Dane Rampe before we started working together. Dane trusted the process, stopped fasting on his days off and tuned in to his subjective metrics like his energy, appetite and performance, which all improved. Over the course of the year, even his external metrics like his skinfolds (a measurement of body fat percentage) improved to the best they had been.

Time-restricted eating sits at the milder end of this spectrum. It focuses on when you eat rather than prolonged fasting, typically within a ten- to 12-hour daytime eating window. This approach still allows the gut an overnight rest and supports your circadian rhythm, while providing more opportunities across the day to meet key nutritional requirements like protein and fibre.[27]

Rather than focus on intermittent fasting, my recommendation is to focus on eating more consistently, improving your diet quality and wholefood intake, and nailing your protein and fibre intake: once that rhythm is in place, more advanced tools like intermittent fasting can be considered and layered in thoughtfully, if they still make sense for your goals.

Eat for your gut

There is another important 'P' word we need to talk about when it comes to your wellbeing and performance. *Plants!*

Plant foods are anything grown in the ground: fruits, vegetables, wholegrains, nuts, seeds, lentils, legumes, herbs and spices. These foods are critical for your gut health because your gut microbiome thrives on them. You can think of these as the favourite foods your good bacteria like to eat. And when you eat these foods, you grow more of the good bacteria, improving the overall ecosystem of your gut.

One of the most influential findings in microbiome research has shown that greater plant diversity in your diet is associated with a more resilient and diverse gut microbiome. Dietary patterns that include around 30 different plant foods across the week consistently outperform those limited to a narrow range of ten or less.[28]

Two clarifications matter here, because I find they tend to cause confusion:

- The target is 30 plant foods per *week*, not per day.
- Those plants come from anything grown in the ground, not just vegetables.

The benefits of focusing on your gut health are far reaching, which is why it is a focus with all of my coaching clients and leadership coaching programs, from elite athletes to executives and everyone in between.

As Olympic sprinter Rohan Browning explains:

> *When I started with Jessica, I was searching for a holistic and detailed approach to nutrition that would adapt with the science. She wanted to really focus on my gut health by increasing colour and diversity and incorporate nutrient timing and periodisation to my eating schedule.*

Tip: Simple swaps for food diversity

The best way to boost up the number of plants you're eating is to look for simple swaps. Rather than just having blueberries in your smoothie, have mixed berries. Instead of having brown rice, have a mixed grain combination. Rather than having almonds, have mixed nuts ... you get the idea.

The role of your gut health

Your gut health is responsible for a lot of important functions, including your digestion, your immunity and your gut microbiome. Around 70 per cent of your immune system lives in your gut, which is home to the gut microbiome.[29] This refers to the environment within the gut that contains trillions of organisms, including bacteria and other microorganisms, both beneficial and harmful. Together, they play a major role in your long-term physical and mental wellbeing.[30]

Your gut is an active system that is in constant communication with your brain, immune system and nervous system via the gut-brain axis. It influences your stress response, hormone regulation, inflammation and how efficiently energy is produced and used.

The way I like to think about the gut is as a manufacturing facility. The gut produces key signalling molecules that influence how we feel and function, including the majority of the body's serotonin (which regulates mood, appetite and sleep) and substantial amounts of dopamine (linked to motivation, reward, focus and drive). This is one of the main ways the gut and brain remain in constant communication with each other.[31]

Basically, what happens in the brain directly affects what happens in the gut and vice versa. This is largely via the vagus nerve and other gut-brain pathways, as shown in figure 4.5 (overleaf).[32] During periods of higher stress, this can show up through changes in your digestion or the onset of gut symptoms, which might not otherwise be there.

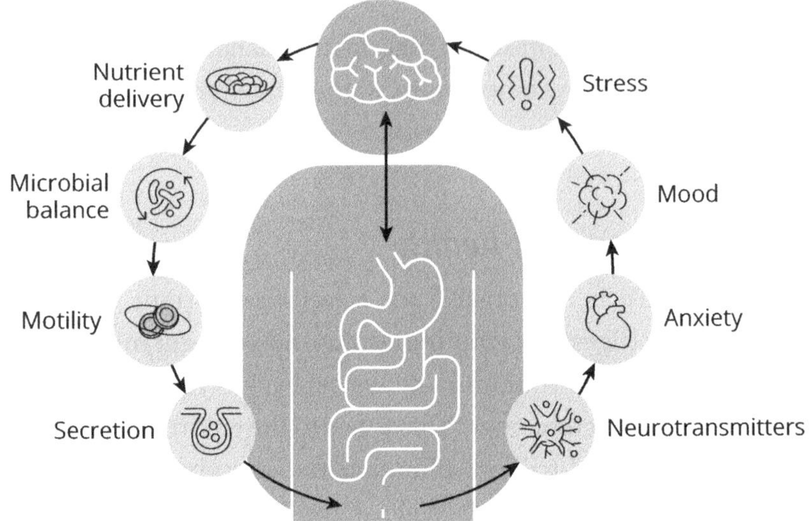

Figure 4.5 *The gut-brain connection*

One of the most common assumptions when digestive symptoms appear is that it must be food, so I need to remove or restrict something. In some instances, this is needed if you have irritable bowel syndrome, but you want to go through this process with an accredited practising dietitian. However, what many people don't realise is that inconsistent intake, repeated restriction and avoidance of foods can, in some cases, actually drive or exacerbate these symptoms, especially when you layer in stress on top.

When it comes to gut health, what you eat is only one part of the picture; non-dietary factors such as stress, nervous system regulation, sleep and exercise also shape gut-brain signalling and symptom severity, which is why effective symptom management almost always involves working on stress and coping, not just what's on your plate.[33]

Where good intentions can go wrong

With all the focus on protein, food manufacturers have responded, and now protein is added to almost everything. But this is where what you eat matters, not just how much protein it contains.

As we discussed on page 70, protein is important to your energy, wellbeing and performance, and so it can be easy to learn this and then just reach for the most convenient type. That might be ready-made meals, protein bars, protein shakes and any other convenient food that has been 'protein boosted'.

But, not all protein foods have been created equally, especially when thinking about the level of processing and how this impacts your gut health. In some cases, these heavily processed protein foods are full of additives and artificial ingredients that place additional stress on your gut.[34]

When we talk about gut health, one of the key areas you want to try and protect is the integrity of your gut wall, known as your *intestinal permeability.*

Intestinal permeability

A healthy gut wall acts as a selective barrier. It allows the right nutrients through while keeping unwanted substances out. When that barrier is compromised, the immune system carries a greater load and low-grade inflammation becomes more likely because more unwanted particles can slip through the gut wall and into your blood stream.[35]

This is one of the reasons why what you eat matters. A diet rich in a variety of plant foods, prebiotics and probiotics supports beneficial gut bacteria, which help maintain and repair your gut barrier wall.

When your good bacteria are well fed with foods rich in prebiotics, they produce short chain fatty acids such as butyrate and propionate, which help strengthen your gut wall by repairing the mucous and directly strengthening your gut barrier integrity.[36]

The way I like to think about the gut wall is through a security lens. When I go out to the Army Barracks to work with the ADF Special Forces, there is a very strict process for me to get on base. I must bring specific identification, be granted access and given a special pass to swipe, which allows me on to the base.

This is how a well-functioning gut wall works. It is selective with who and what it lets through; it only lets through the right things under the right conditions.

A leaky gut wall is the opposite. It is as if the army barracks' security system and boom gate malfunctioned and it started letting anyone in, without checks or control. This would be a significant security breach, and it is not something your immune system wants either.

Favourite foods for your microbiome

Here is a summary of the favourite foods for your microbiome:

- *Prebiotic* foods are fibres, including resistant starch, that your body can't digest but your gut microbes can, helping them grow and produce beneficial compounds like short chain fatty acids. Examples include onion, garlic, leeks,

asparagus, oats, barley, legumes, nuts, seeds, apples, slightly green bananas, cooked and cooled potatoes, rice and pasta.
- *Probiotics* and fermented foods that contain live cultures and/or fermentation processes can support a healthy gut environment. Examples include yoghurt with live cultures, kefir, some cottage cheeses, sauerkraut, kimchi, miso, tempeh and sourdough bread.

Piecing together the protein and plant protocol

This is a simple framework to bring together what we have covered in the protein and plant sections.

For women: 30 | 30 | 30

- 30 grams of protein per meal
- 30 grams of fibre per day (minimum)
- 30 different plant foods per week

For men: 40–50 | 30 | 30

- 40 to 50 grams of protein per meal
- 30 grams of fibre per day (minimum)
- 30 different plant foods per week

Nutrition periodisation: adjust intake to output

If you have made it this far and this section feels like your opportunity to elevate your nutrition rhythm, you are already doing a great job!

Nutrition periodisation may sound more complicated than what it is but it really just refers to the practice of matching what you eat to your demands, which is largely based on how active you are. Some days you require more when you are more active, other days less when you are less active.

It is really easy to have a flat-line approach with your nutrition—you eat the same meals most days and weeks as a default process. It's one less thing to think about. But, if your days have different demands, this approach creates a mismatch between what you are doing and what you need.

Nutrition is often thought of in terms of what needs to be subtracted or removed. It might be 'I am cutting carbs' or 'I am reducing fat' or 'I need to reduce my portions'.

If you think back to how this chapter started, the issue with many common nutrition approaches is that they disrupt rhythm and remove key elements. That inconsistency is exactly what makes appetite harder to regulate and energy harder to sustain.

Nutrition periodisation works because it preserves structure while allowing flexibility, and it is customised to your life, because you:

- Retain the overall consistency of your meals and snacks. This includes when you start eating, when you stop, the spacing between meals and whether you include snacks. Timing stays consistent.
- Retain all four elements at every meal. Protein, carbohydrates, colours and healthy fats should always be present. When you adjust your intake based on output, the variables that adjust are carbohydrates and colours. Protein and fats should stay stable, every meal, every day.

- Retain the overall volume of food. Meal size matters. Rather than eating larger or smaller meals, you want to have a consistent volume of food, but you adjust some of the ratios on the plate.
- Adjust carbohydrates and colours based on activity. On more active days, you increase carbohydrates and, to accommodate, reduce the colours element slightly. On less active days, you reduce the amount of carbohydrates and increase your colours to create the same volume. Protein and healthy fats remain consistent regardless of your activity levels for the day. This consistency is key for appetite regulation and stable energy.[37]

The way I like to communicate this point is with plate ratios because a picture says a thousand words.

Why plate ratios work

Plate ratios provide a visual, intuitive way to adjust intake in real time that doesn't require anything overly complex. Here is a diagram of the three key plate ratios.

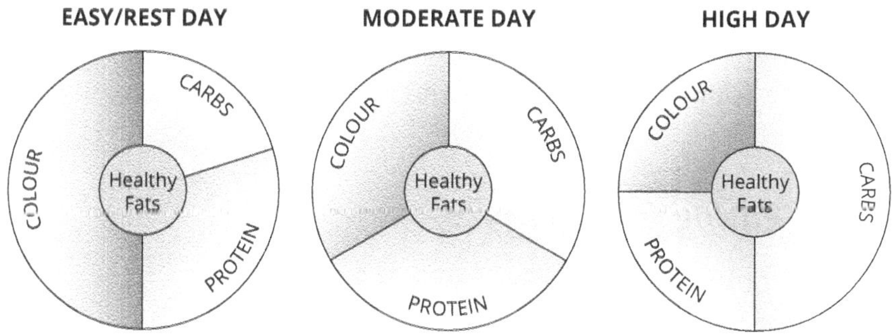

Figure 4.6 ***Periodising intake (with plate ratios)***

If you look at the diagrams, you will notice:

- Protein: always takes up a quarter to a third of the plate.
- Healthy fats: always take up the same amount (approximately a tablespoon).
- The carbohydrates and colours vary the most: when you have more colours, you have fewer carbohydrates, and vice versa.

In most instances, low- and medium-output days will make up the majority of your week. High-output days are only needed when demands are high, such as if you're training for a marathon or triathlon, if you're an elite athlete or if you have an active teenager who seems to be eating you out of house and home.

If you under-fuel on high-demand days, this can lead to you having more fatigue, more cravings, poor recovery and disrupted sleep. It also creates a flow-on effect, where you feel much hungrier later that day or the next. Whenever an athlete would tell me they were 'starving on their day off', I always knew this meant they had under-fuelled the day before.

The plate ratio concept is nutrition periodisation in a practical framework. It allows you to take things to the next level, but only once the foundations have been laid. The order of this chapter is deliberate, it is sequential and it is designed to be a tailored roadmap. Start with the habit or behaviour that presents your first opportunity to elevate your nutrition rhythm and then layer from there.

Tip: Eating for energy

With nutrition periodisation:

- All four elements (protein, carbohydrates, colours and healthy fats) are present.

- Protein and healthy fats remain consistent for all meals on all days.
- Carbohydrates and colours adjust based on your needs.
- The volume of your meal should always be consistent, it's the elements that adjust to match your needs.

Hydrate the CEO

Last, but certainly not least, we need to talk about hydration. When I say hydrate the CEO, I am not talking about your boss. I am talking about the most important decision-maker in your body: your brain.

Every thought, every choice, every reaction, every physiological function, every moment of focus or fatigue is directed by your brain. And one of the simplest, most overlooked ways most of us undermine our performance is hydration.

Your brain is approximately 75 per cent water. Let that land! This is why even mild dehydration has an impact on your cognitive performance, which can include:

- your focus dropping
- your mental fatigue increasing
- tasks feeling harder than they should.

Research shows that even mild dehydration of just 1 to 2 per cent of body weight is enough to impair attention, working memory and decision-making, while increasing mental fatigue.[38] All of this can happen before the cue most of us rely on strikes—thirst!

You also lose 0.5 to 1 litre of fluid every night through breathing and sweating. That means most of us are already waking mildly dehydrated.[39] If you don't proactively start hydrating in the morning, that deficit is carried throughout your day.

If the first thing you drink in the morning is a coffee, you hit the gym and sweat, and you don't think about drinking anything until you get thirsty mid-morning, it's no wonder your body and brain are dehydrated!

Hydration is commonly treated as a reactive behaviour. Most of us wait until we're thirsty to drink. We also drink until our thirst is quenched, which can mean a whole bottle is drunk in seconds or minutes. Like your meals, you ideally want to evenly spread it across the day.

I saw this clearly during my time working in elite sport. One of my roles was to test the athletes' hydration status on main training days. That involved exactly what you are thinking—collecting urine samples and measuring them with an instrument called a refractometer. Glamorous!

Even among elite athletes who are paid to perform, the majority arrived at training dehydrated. If dehydration is common in elite environments with full support teams, it is almost guaranteed in everyday life unless you are proactive, intentional and strategic with it.

Tip: Hydrate before you caffeinate

Rather than starting your morning with coffee, start with a glass of water or electrolytes. Ideally, drink that first, but if that sounds too hard, at least consume the water and your coffee at the same time. This is to build non-negotiable behaviours that support your energy and performance across the day.

What's the deal with electrolytes?

Electrolytes refer to sodium, magnesium and potassium. They play critical roles in nerve signalling, muscle contraction and fluid balance. The main electrolyte to pay attention to is sodium. When we sweat, this is the primary electrolyte we lose. And if we eat well, largely whole foods, we also tend to consume less sodium, as it is found predominantly in packaged and processed foods.

Sodium has a really important role in fluid balance. This is not just how much we drink, but how much we retain. If you are active and eat mostly whole foods, you might like to experiment with starting your morning with electrolytes.

If you struggle to drink enough water, adding electrolytes can also help increase overall fluid intake. One brand that I have worked closely with is Hyro.

Like nutrition, hydration is a behaviour that compounds. When it becomes a non-negotiable, proactive behaviour with a rhythm across the day, rather than a reactive afterthought, the impact on energy, focus and performance adds up quickly! Give it a try.

Eat better to sleep better

All your rhythms are closely connected, in particular nutrition and sleep. The way you eat influences how you sleep, and how you sleep influences how you eat.

From a nutrition perspective, how and when you eat plays a key role in how well you sleep. Late, heavy or large meals place additional demand on your digestive system at a time when your body is trying to downregulate and restore. Data from WHOOP shows this can delay the time it takes you to get to sleep, reduce the time you spend in your most restorative phases and impair your overall recovery overnight.[40] This is one of the many reasons why eating with rhythm matters. Not just for daytime energy, but for how well you recover at night.

Many of the strategies you have been introduced to in this chapter support you getting a good night's sleep, but here's a summary to help you eat better to sleep better:

- A high-protein first meal stabilises appetite and energy.
- Protein pulsing across the day reduces cravings and supports focus.
- Consistent meal timing avoids long gaps or large late meals.
- Meals rich in fibre slow digestion and support gut health.
- Adequate hydration supports cognitive function and reduces perceived fatigue.

Putting this into practice

Nutrition is a science, but eating is a behaviour, which is why you need a personalised strategy to help you consistently execute your nutrition rhythm. If you love spending Sunday afternoons grocery shopping and meal prepping—great. If you don't, then let's find a strategy that will fit your life.

Here are some strategies that might help you be more consistent with your nutrition rhythm.

1. Online grocery shopping

This is one of my go-to strategies. Most major supermarkets and many local butchers and providers now offer online ordering. You can shop weekly, set up a recurring order or simply repeat a previous shop in your account. A recurring order does not mean eating the same foods forever. Think around 60 to 70 per cent consistent. Your weekly staples such as eggs, bread, milk, yoghurt stay the same. Then rotate fruit, vegetables and protein sources each week to maintain diversity with minimal effort.

2. Partially prepared meals

If the end of the week is where things fall apart, this could be a great option for you. Some providers have part of the meal, rather than a full meal, such as the protein component, which is often the most time consuming. If you have this part sorted, it can significantly reduce prep time. Two of the companies I use and recommend often for this are Dineamic and The Dinner Ladies.

3. Meal kits

Meal kits can work well if you still want to cook but want the process of ordering or buying done for you. While these can be great time-saving options, you do want to be selective, as some options can be carbohydrate heavy and light on protein or vegetables. Now you know what to look for (such as 20 to 40 grams of protein per serve), use this knowledge to make the best selections, or upgrade the meal kit you have with a side salad or frozen vegetables.

4. Ready-made meals

There is a place for these, but it is important to know they are not all created equal. When choosing these options, look for ones with short ingredients lists and check the amount of protein and servings of vegetables. Again, you can boost up the vegetables with a side salad or some extra vegetables if they are lacking.

5. Pay for someone to prep your meals

I realise this is not a strategy available to everyone—personally, it's on my goals list for 'one day'! I do have some clients and athletes who have a chef prepare their meals or some of their meals. At face value this might seem like a more expensive option, or not possible, but if you are regularly eating out or using Uber Eats, it could be worth doing a cost comparison.

Tip: Easy pantry staples to elevate your nutrition

Keep these foods on hand to make nutrition easier and instantly lift meal quality:

- yoghurt and frozen fruit such as berries for smoothies or quick breakfasts
- pre-washed salad mixes to add volume and fibre with zero prep
- frozen vegetables for fast, reliable vegetable intake
- tinned lentils and legumes for protein, fibre and gut health support
- mixed nuts or seeds to add healthy fats, texture and satiety.

A word on supplements

Supplements are something I regularly use with my clients from elite athletes to CEOs to everyday people, but there are some specific conditions to this.

They are the icing on the cake

Supplements do not form the foundation of the nutrition rhythm; they are implemented once all the other strategies here have been covered. To give them the best chance of having an effect, your fundamentals need to be in place first, particularly consistent routines and supportive daily behaviours. This means you take a food first approach.

Choose wisely

When choosing supplements, I always recommend using products that are third-party batch tested through programs such as HASTA or Informed Sport. Elite athletes must consume supplements with this level of testing, and for everyone else, this brings a level of safety and quality, so we know we are only consuming what it says on the label. Supplements are one of the most cross-contaminated product categories, with roughly one-third of non-batch-tested sports supplements testing positive to prohibited substances.[41]

In Chapter 7, I share a few of the sleep supplements I use with clients or recommend in this space. Other than these, there are only a handful of supplements that I recommend for most people, and, even then, this is highly individualised depending on their lifestyle, goals, medical history and, most importantly, their pathology. Some supplements you might like to explore include:

- Omega 3 fatty acids to optimise omega-3 index, anti-inflammatory properties, brain health and healthy ageing.
- Vitamin C, which should be used as part of an immune protocol, not as an everyday, year-round supplement.
- Zinc should also be used as part of an immune protocol, and not necessarily as something that you take every day.
- Vitamin D for when you are deficient or aiming to optimise your vitamin D status.
- Magnesium (discussed in more detail in Chapter 7) to aid in sleep and recovery.
- Creatine (discussed in more detail in Chapter 7) has broad benefits, including physical performance and cognitive function. Emerging evidence shows that it can help buffer some of the performance and cognitive impacts of short-term sleep deprivation.

Activity

To get clear on what your nutrition rhythm looks like right now, reflect on these questions:

- How many meals and snacks do you need to have on a weekday to feel your best?
- How many meals and snacks do you need to have on the weekend to feel your best?
- Write out your meal and snack rhythm. Aim for a consistent 'eating window' for each meal (30 to 60 minutes) so you keep a consistent rhythm.

Conclusion

Eating is one of the only behaviours, other than sleeping and breathing, that you do every single day. When it comes to improving your energy, wellbeing and performance, both today and in the future, your nutrition rhythm is one of the most powerful levers that is totally within your control.

When it comes to creating or elevating your nutrition rhythm, start at the front of this chapter and work on the behaviours that you can improve. By doing this you will truly leverage the full potential of this important rhythm.

Remember, when it comes to your nutrition rhythm, what you eat and how you eat are equally important, while also factoring what you need and the nuances, such as the quality of your food and the need for diversity.

The best bit, elevating your nutrition rhythm is about focusing on what you should be having, rather than focusing on restricting foods. When your nutrition rhythm becomes more predictable, your appetite and cravings are easier to manage, your energy is steadier and decision-making becomes less reactive.

Chapter Five

Exercise — Exercise creates energy

How many times have you skipped a workout because you *'didn't have the energy'*?

It's one of the biggest traps. We tell ourselves we need energy to exercise, when exercise is one of the fastest ways to create it.

Aside from the immediate energy boost exercise gives you, it also sets off a cascade of beneficial physiological processes, which is why it has earned the phrase 'exercise is medicine'.

There's also been research showing that when you start a structured exercise program, you are more likely to improve your diet at the same time.[42] And when you're exercising regularly, it also improves your sleep. You can see how interconnected these five rhythms are, and how much you can leverage one to gain momentum with less effort. Green flags! This is exactly the kind of compounding effect we are trying to harness as you build your operating system.

When movement becomes part of how you operate, your identity, this can help reduce the amount of friction you're met with, or the amount of motivation you need, to get moving. In his book *Atomic*

Habits, James Clear describes how behaviours tied to our identity require less motivation and are more likely to stick because they become an expression of who we are rather than something we must force.

Another narrative that may speak to you is *'I just don't like exercise'*. If this is you, the starting point is finding something you do not actively resist. Remember, we want the path of least resistance, especially while you are trying to start or become more consistent with something. So, if the idea of going for a run is an absolute no, what about a swim or a cycle class? If you don't want to go to the gym on your own to do weights, could you work with a personal trainer while you build confidence and momentum? If all else fails, can you go for a walk with a friend on the weekend or on your lunch break?

This chapter will walk through the different types of exercise and why they matter, but if this rhythm is the one you struggle with the most, it's important to remember this: *something is always better than nothing.* Any movement counts when starting out or trying to establish your rhythm because consistency beats intensity.

Sometimes the block is not exercise itself, but the meaning attached to it. If movement has been framed purely around how you look, that may not mean enough to you to sustain it, especially in demanding seasons of life.

Instead, maybe something more meaningful will be what exercise gives you, such as how it makes you feel afterward. If this is coming up for you, maybe see if you can start to observe the difference between the days you move and the days you don't:

- Is your mood better?
- Do you manage stress more easily?

- Do you sleep more deeply?
- Do you feel more patient, more focused or more like yourself?

Personally, the answer for me is a big *yes* to all of those.

For me, exercise is a non-negotiable for my mood. Even a short walk changes how I show up at work and how I show up with my daughter. On days I have not slept as well as I would like (and there are plenty of them), I am often tempted to stay in bed — and have at times. But I also know that when I stay in bed, I don't go back to sleep, and it makes me feel worse. Then I'll often skip movement altogether, and the outcome of that? I am snappier, less focused and far less productive across the day.

So, when I ask myself whether I want to feel more energised, focused and be in a better mood *or* be snappier, less focused and less productive, the decision is an easy one. Get up and move! If you struggle to find motivation to move, this kind of reflection or reframe might be the missing link for you too.

I was speaking to a group of senior leaders at an off-site when one of the CEOs shared that, for years, exercise felt like an obligation to her. She resisted it, struggled to stay consistent and never enjoyed it. That changed when someone close to her was diagnosed with a degenerative neurological condition. Exercise stopped being about appearance and it became about the mental benefits, preserving function, independence, and the quality of life. Her relationship with exercise shifted almost overnight.

If you're waiting to start exercising more regularly once you feel better or 'have the time', this is your sign to rewrite that narrative and find your exercise rhythm. Aside from being rewarded with a multitude of benefits with your mood, your focus, your energy, you are also paying dividends to the future version of you. Exercise is one of the strongest levers we have for protecting our long-term health. Our cardiorespiratory fitness, strength and muscle mass are among the most powerful predictors of longevity, independence and quality of life as we age, and exercise is a core driver for all of those.

If this is where you get stuck, the answer is not about finding more time, it is about *making* time. This is where the operating system you are building will help you big time. When you understand your rhythms and see how this feeds into your energy, and how it helps you show up consistently, it will become something easier to navigate. The trick is being persistent and starting with what you can consistently manage and build on over time.

Also, I am sure if you did a time audit you could find some extra time to move by cutting down on one less Netflix episode or the mindless scrolling in the evening—or even stopping the snooze in the morning. There are plenty of options once we look for solutions and opportunities.

With all your rhythms, being consistent and proactive is important. But with your exercise rhythm, it may work better for you if you have some flexibility built in, like I have had to do for this season of life. Sure, you might have your preferred time of day to exercise—maybe it's the morning, lunchtime or the afternoon—but if that isn't always possible, how can you adapt? Alternatively, maybe it means starting to wake up earlier than you have been. This might be difficult for the first few days or week, but over time you adjust.

For me, as a lion chronotype (see page 52 for a refresher), mornings are my preferred time to exercise. I am happy to walk or do yoga later in the day, but more intense training works best earlier. But, in this current season of life with my one-year-old, that is not always possible. I often need to coordinate schedules with my partner, which means some sessions happen mid-morning or at lunchtime. I struggled with this at first. I skipped sessions, I made excuses or would get stuck in analysis paralysis. Eventually, once I accepted this is the current season I am in and when I attached the meaning back to my mood and how I show up with my daughter, this helped me find my new exercise rhythm and accept that something is better than nothing. This is the operating system I am working with right now, and I feel so much better on the days I move!

> ***Tip: The exercise-energy reframe***
>
> Repeat after me: exercise is not something I do once I have energy, it is one of the fastest ways to create it.

Exercise is medicine

If pharmaceutical companies could bottle what exercise does for us, it would be the most prescribed drug in the world. Exercise changes how you function now, and it influences how you age. The effects are immediate and long-lasting. Exercise works on two timelines at once.

Within minutes of starting to exercise, muscle contractions release chemical messengers that communicate with the brain and nervous system. These neurotransmitters enhance mood and motivation, and increase focus as well as the blood flow to your brain. Thinking becomes clearer, decision-making easier and emotional control stronger. This is why even a short walk or a gym session can change the direction of your day. I am sure if you've ever wanted to skip a gym class or a workout, but you went, you didn't regret it because you felt better after![43]

At the same time, exercise is shaping your future self. Regular exercise is one of the most important factors of long-term health and longevity. Your cardiorespiratory fitness, often assessed by your VO_2 max, reflects how well your body can cope with physical and metabolic stress.[44] Strength and muscle mass help reduce the risk of injury, illness and loss of independence, and higher muscle mass is strongly associated with better cognitive and brain health in older age.[45]

What exercise does for you today

- Lifts energy and mood: Exercise increases neurotransmitters linked to motivation and emotional regulation.
- Sharpens thinking and focus: Increased blood flow and neuroplasticity support clearer thinking, creativity and better decision-making.
- Reduces stress in real time: Exercise helps metabolise stress hormones and provides a physical outlet for mental load.
- Creates momentum: When your energy improves, your focus is sharpened and the rest of the day becomes easier as you move from one task to the next.

What exercise does for future you

- Protects long-term health and longevity: Regular exercise is strongly associated with lower risk of premature death.
- Builds cardiorespiratory fitness: Higher fitness reflects greater physiological resilience and is linked to longer health span.
- Preserves strength and muscle mass: Muscle supports metabolic health, injury prevention and independence. It also combats age-related strength and muscle decline (sarcopenia).
- Supports brain health: Exercise is associated with lower risk of cognitive decline and supports long-term brain function.

I don't know about you, but I want behaviours that help me show up better now and protect future me too. Exercise does both.

Your exercise portfolio

Have you ever thought *'Should I be doing cardio or strength training?'* Much like a share portfolio where you want diversification, exercise is similar. It's not which one should you do, it's *both*!

Together, different types of cardiovascular and resistance training support two of the most important components to our energy, resilience and long-term health: our cardiorespiratory fitness and our muscle mass.

Here's the rundown on why you want to focus on strength training, cardio and add in some balance and flexibility work.

Strength training

This is one of the most important investments you can make in your future health.

Strength training, also known as resistance training, is any exercise where your muscles contract against an external resistance. When you do this, you create tiny amounts of stress and breakdown of muscle fibres, as your body repairs that damage, the muscles adapt and become stronger. There is a wide range of exercises in this category, including weights, machines, bands and your body weight.

Muscle is metabolically active tissue that helps regulate your blood sugar, supports joint health, protects against injury and underpins how resilient you feel day to day. From midlife onwards, muscle and bone loss accelerate unless you actively work against it with a combination of strength training and nutrition intervention (which we covered in Chapter 4) to support this.

When your muscles contract during strength training, they release signalling proteins called myokines that act as chemical messengers. They travel through the bloodstream to influence other organs, including the brain. Some of these myokines, such as irisin and brain-derived neurotrophic factor (BDNF), are involved in supporting neuroplasticity, learning and memory, which is one reason strength training is consistently linked with better cognitive outcomes as we age.[46]

For women, particularly through perimenopause and beyond, this becomes even more important. Hormonal shifts, largely the decline in oestrogen, accelerate the rate of muscle loss and blunt the body's anabolic response to both protein and training, contributing to wider metabolic change. Less muscle means less metabolic support and potentially fewer of these beneficial signalling effects. Maintaining or even gaining lean mass through structured resistance training is, therefore, one of the most powerful ways to support both metabolic and cognitive health in this phase.[47]

A quick note on Pilates. Pilates is excellent for core strength, posture, balance and body awareness; however most Pilates classes do not provide the kind of progressively heavier loading recommended in resistance training guidelines to slow or reverse age-related loss of muscle mass and strength, so it should be seen as a complement to, not a replacement for, dedicated strength training.

What does 'enough' strength training look like?

Preserving and building muscle mass means working the major muscle groups two to three times per week, doing two to three sets of six to 12 controlled repetitions per exercise, with a load that feels challenging by the last few reps. The key is progressive overload, which means gradually increasing the weight, reps or difficulty over time so the muscles keep getting a strong reason to adapt.[48]

A note on safety and support

If you have never lifted weights or have medical conditions, it is important not to jump straight into heavy lifting on your own. Starting with lighter loads, learning good technique and, where possible, getting guidance from a qualified exercise professional can reduce injury risk and help you build confidence and strength step by step.

Sarcopenia and age-related changes

When we are younger, our muscles respond well to things like strength training and eating enough protein, pulsed across the day. These signals tell the body to build and maintain muscle (through the process of muscle protein synthesis) while limiting muscle breakdown.

As we get older, the response becomes less effective. Muscles stop reacting as strongly to the same signals (anabolic resistance). The result is that muscle is built more slowly and broken down more easily.[49]

Body composition changes in perimenopause and menopause

Research has shown that women go through a short, intense phase of bone loss around menopause, with bone density at the spine and hip dropping the fastest in the years just before and after their final period. It also showed that even when body weight hardly changes, women typically lose muscle and gain abdominal fat across this transition. These shifts in body composition are linked to less favourable blood sugar control and blood fat profiles.[50]

The good news is that with targeted intervention, primarily well-designed resistance training and adequate protein and nutrition, as discussed in Chapter 4, these changes can be slowed substantially and even improved upon.

Cardiovascular training

Cardiovascular training, or cardio, targets your cardiorespiratory fitness, which is how well your heart, lungs and blood vessels deliver oxygen to working muscles during physical activity. Regular cardiovascular training strengthens the heart, increases the amount of blood pumped with each beat, and improves your ability to transport and use oxygen, allowing the body to move, work and recover more efficiently. Examples of cardio include running, swimming, cycling, rowing, dancing, tennis, netball, football, basketball and surfing.

And just as these activities can look very different, they can also feel very different—from easy conversational efforts to all out sprints, which is where the idea of heart rate training zones comes in. Of the five commonly described zones, two sit at opposite ends of the intensity range: zone 2 and zone 5.

Zone 2 (low to moderate exercise) and zone 5 (near maximal, very hard cardio in short bursts) drive distinct physiological adaptations, which is why they form the foundation of most evidence-based cardiovascular programs. This is about being deliberate with intensity and not just sitting in the middle; pushing harder but training smarter.

Lower intensity (zone 2)

Zone 2 cardio improves how well your body produces and uses energy, so everyday activities start to feel easier when this aerobic base is in place. Examples include brisk walking, cycling or steady swimming at about 60 to 70 per cent of your maximum heart rate. The litmus test here is that you should be able to carry out a conversation, although it may not be particularly comfortable, you can do it.

Higher intensity (zone 5)

Zone 5 cardio places a direct demand on the heart and lungs, pushing you to near maximal effort for a short period of time. It typically involves brief intervals at around 90 to 100 per cent of your maximum heart rate, followed by full recovery.

To start this might look like 15 to 30 seconds of hill sprints, rowing, battle ropes or assault bike, followed by one to two minutes of full recovery. It can also look like slightly longer intervals, often referred to as VO_2 max training (more on this on page 120), which usually means working at around 85 to 95 per cent of maximum heart rate for three to five minutes. It's tough, and you don't need to start here if this is new to your exercise rhythm.

A recent study showed that even small amounts of incidental movement, meaning activity built into daily life, can significantly reduce cardiovascular risk. Just one minute of vigorous incidental movement delivered a similar benefit to around three minutes of moderate incidental activity, reinforcing that short, higher-effort bouts can have an outsized impact on long-term cardiovascular health.[51]

In practical terms, this often looks like a combination of easier, conversational-pace movement and brief periods of higher effort. A consistent base, paired with brief moments of intensity, gives you the most benefit for the time you have and most efficiently builds the capacity that protects your health over the long run.

Balance and mobility

Balance and mobility are the quiet contributors that rarely get attention until they are suddenly missed. They support movement confidence, reduce injury risk and protect independence as you age.

Balance and mobility work does not need to be fancy or time consuming. At home, it might be a few minutes of standing on one leg while you brush your teeth, slow squats to a chair, heel-to-toe walking down the hallway or some light foam rolling. Otherwise, you might prefer to go to a Pilates, yoga or barre class. If you follow a strength program, you may have this box ticked in there. For me, I have some incorporated in the gym sessions I do as some prehabilitation, and then I also use a foam roller (most nights) for five to ten minutes while I watch TV. If I miss it for a few days, I feel it!

Balance and mobility work is kind of like future insurance for your joints and stability—like WD-40 but for your body.

How much do I need?

Australia's national physical activity guidelines recommend adults aim to be active on most days of the week and accumulate a weekly dose of movement that supports long-term health and resilience, which for adults aged 18 to 64, looks like:

- 150 to 300 minutes (2½ to 5 hours) of moderate-intensity activity, or 75 to 150 minutes (1¼ to 2½ hours) of vigorous activity, or an equivalent mix of both per week
- muscle-strengthening activities, such as resistance work, weights or functional strength exercises, done on at least two days each week
- sedentary time matters too: breaking up long periods of sitting is recommended because uninterrupted sitting is linked with poorer metabolic outcomes.[52]

The guidelines also state that doing any physical activity is better than doing none. If you do no physical activity right now, you can slowly build up to the recommended amount, which brings us to our next point.

Something is better than nothing

One of the biggest barriers to movement is all-or-nothing thinking. If it cannot be done 'properly', it does not get done at all. This might be you don't have time to get to your favourite class, or you can't get your normal 30- or 45-minute run or walk in, so you don't go. The better alternative would be adjusting what you can do to the time you have available. If you only have 15 minutes, a 15-minute walk or run is better than none.

What we now know is that there really is no minimum amount of time or dose for benefit—it all counts! This is amazing news, and great for helping us fit our exercise rhythm into our operating system. This means that a ten-minute YouTube circuit counts, a short walk between meetings counts, ten air squats between each call counts. They all count!

Even the smallest exercise 'dose' beats zero every time. If you find you are getting stuck because you can't do what you would like, lower the bar. Remember, this is about starting with the exercise rhythm you can sustain on your busiest weeks, not just your best. Once something is in place, you can build on it.

On the other hand, you also don't want to go from zero to 100. If you have not trained in months or been inconsistent, and then 'kick start' things back up with an attempt at daily classes or back-to-back PT sessions, there is a good chance this will become unsustainable, or worst-case, lead to an injury. The constant stopping and starting when it comes to exercise and injury is called the boom-to-bust cycle that you want to avoid.

Tip: Kick-start your exercise rhythm

If you are struggling to get into a regular exercise rhythm, here are some ways that might help you find your rhythm:

- Book your exercise classes ahead of time — and if you cancel, you have to pay a fee.
- Exercise with a friend for accountability.
- Put your clothes out the night before — this is a must for me!
- Block exercise in your diary like any other important meeting.
- Focus on exercise snacks.

Exercise snacks

You already know I love a good food snack from Chapter 4, but this is the other kind I'm a big fan of: exercise snacks!

Exercise snacks are, ultimately, short, intentional bursts of movement you sprinkle through the day. Nothing fancy, just movement that fits into real life that delivers results. Green flags!

Most of our days are built around sitting: meetings, screens, cars, planes, couches. The problem is, because of this, we often sit for too long without breaking it up, and, over time, that starts to chip away at energy, focus and metabolic health, so much so, that it has even earned the phrase 'sitting is the new smoking'.

The good news is that short bouts of movement for even one to three minutes can offset this prolonged sitting with a range of benefits (see table 5.1, which is adapted from the study by Alexe et al.[53]).

Table 5.1 *The benefits of exercise snacks*

Health domain	Outcomes from exercise snacks
Metabolic health	↓ post-meal blood glucose, ↓ insulin, ↑glucose tolerance
Cardiovascular function	↓ blood pressure
Musculoskeletal fitness	↑ lower-limb strength
Cognitive performance	↑ alertness, ↓ fatigue, ↑ mood, ↑ acute cognition
Behavioural adherence	≥ 80 per cent adherence to sustainable daily integration

So, what are some examples of exercise snacks? They could look like:

- a brisk walk between meetings
- taking the stairs instead of the lift
- ten air squats, push-ups, burpees or star jumps every 30 to 60 minutes
- 30 seconds of sit-to-stands from your office chair every hour.

I understand some of these might be easier for you to do at home than in the office, but if that's the case, taking the stairs is a great option, or utilising a space all to yourself like a meeting room.

A 2024 meta-analysis of 27 randomised trials found that short, frequent bouts of movement significantly improved cardiorespiratory fitness, reduced body fat and lowered blood pressure, making exercise snacks a time-efficient option for busy lives.[54] The bottom line? Little and often beats nothing.

We need to move more and sit less

Today, more than half of Australian adults do not meet basic movement recommendations. Most people move too little and sit for too long. While life today is built around sitting at work, commuting, screens and routines, human beings have biologically been designed to *move*.

The issue is not *only* that we are not exercising enough, but that we are sitting for too long. Hours of sitting without breaking it up negatively affects metabolic health and is associated with a higher risk of type 2 diabetes and cardiovascular disease, even in people who train regularly.

That is why the message is not just *move more*. It is *move more* and *sit less*.

Here are some ways you can do this in your day:

- stand up during calls
- take walking meetings
- get off the train or bus one stop early
- walk between meetings
- take the stairs
- park further away.

Your body and brain respond best to regular movement spread across waking hours, not long stretches of stillness followed by a single burst of effort, and it all starts by sprinkling more movement intentionally into your day and building a consistent exercise rhythm.

A note on pain, niggles and injuries

Being in pain is no fun. If exercise has dropped for you because of pain, injury or a past bad experience, I get it—with my own share of niggles and injuries over the years, I really do. But what you want to avoid is stopping all together. Instead, this is where adapting and getting the right support matters.

Depending on what you're managing, you might benefit from working with one or more of the following:

- physiotherapist: to assess pain or injury, guide rehabilitation and help you return to movement safely and confidently
- exercise physiologist: to design and progress exercise around injury, pain or medical conditions, with a strong focus on long-term health and function
- strength coach: to rebuild strength, resilience and capacity once pain is under control, and reduce the risk of future injury through better movement and loading
- experienced personal trainer: to support consistency, correct technique and appropriate progression, particularly if you need accountability while working within physical limits.

As the saying goes, 'if you don't use it, you lose it'. This is the principle of reversibility, and it is why continuing to move, in a modified and intentional way, is so important.

Testing and metrics for my data people

Have you heard the saying 'what gets measured gets managed'?

The longevity movement that is happening right now is shining a light on the value of proactive baseline testing. When you know where things sit while you're feeling well, it's much easier to spot meaningful changes over time. Proactive baseline testing can also reveal blind spots or weaknesses you might otherwise miss, and point towards targeted interventions or areas that deserve more attention.

You do not need to track everything, but there are a few numbers that are helpful for you to know—some of them you need to do externally, some can be tracked with a wearable which was discussed in Chapter 2.

VO_2 max testing

VO_2 max measures maximal oxygen uptake and aerobic capacity. It is one of the strongest predictors we have of long-term health and longevity. Many wearables estimate VO_2 max, but having it measured formally gives you a true baseline that you can compare against over time if you choose.

DEXA scan

A DEXA scan measures your body composition, which includes your muscle mass, fat mass and bone density. It is considered the gold standard of imaging for body composition and is useful for understanding both health and long-term health risk. I recommend an annual DEXA scan to monitor how you're tracking, or every six months if you are trying to change your body composition.

Grip strength test

Grip strength is one of the simplest and most powerful indicators of overall strength and future health. It reflects your muscle mass, total body strength and how well your body is ageing. You can test it a few ways, including a dead hang where you hold a pull-up bar for as long as you can, or a farmer's carry where you walk about 40 metres with heavy kettlebells or dumbbells. Dr Peter Attia often talks about this on *The Drive* podcast, calling grip strength a 'canary in the coal mine' for ageing because it tracks muscle loss and metabolic decline earlier than many lab markers as it's a proxy for total body strength and muscle mass.[55]

There are also useful metrics you can track yourself with a wearable if you choose:

Resting heart rate

Resting heart rate can act as a baseline marker of cardiovascular fitness and overall load, with trends over time being far more meaningful than single readings. It can also be a helpful marker for illness or stress when it increases before visible signs and symptoms appear.

Heart rate variability (HRV)

HRV reflects how your nervous system is coping with stress and recovery and is best used to notice patterns. It can be helpful to see behaviours that are supportive when your HRV is higher (such as consistent sleep, adequate hydration and time outdoors), and behaviours that might be causing additional strain on your body (such as alcohol, late nights or accumulated stress), causing your HRV to lower. I've had many people shocked by how significantly even 'a few drinks' impacts their HRV.

Movement trends

Movement trends, such as steps or active minutes, can help highlight whether long periods of sitting are creeping back into your day, or how you are going with your exercise rhythm. The key with any metric is context. One number on one day means very little. Patterns over weeks and months are where real insight lives.

Let's debunk a few myths

The wellbeing space is crowded with conflicting advice about what actually drives results. Here are a few common misconceptions around exercise and body composition that are worth setting the record straight on.

Myth 1: I have a slow metabolism

In most cases, your metabolism is not broken or slow, but you may be under-muscled. The biggest driver of your resting metabolic rate is your muscle mass, as muscle is the most metabolically active tissue. The more you have, the more energy your body requires at rest. As muscle declines, metabolic rate slows with it.

This is why the most effective ways to support metabolic health is strength training and adequate nutrition, particularly sufficient protein. Resistance training sends a clear signal to the body to preserve and build muscle.

The goal is, therefore, not to 'rev up' your metabolism with more cardio or aggressive restriction. It is to protect and build the tissue that keeps metabolism robust in the first place: your muscle mass!

Myth 2: You need 10 000 steps a day

Don't get me wrong, steps are great and most people would benefit from doing more each day, but the 10 000-step target did not come from health research. It originated from a Japanese marketing campaign in the 1960s for a pedometer, which translates to '10 000-step meter'.

More recent research suggests meaningful health benefits, including lower mortality and improved cardiovascular health, occur at around 7000 to 8000 steps per day. Beyond ~10000 steps, that return begins to plateau for most outcomes.[56]

Steps still matter. They are an accessible way to increase daily movement and reduce sedentary time. Consistency and overall movement across the week matter far more than hitting a single day or a one off target.

Myth 3: Fasted cardio is best

Remember Jeff from Chapter 2? Fasted training is not inherently better. It depends on the purpose of the session.

For short, low-intensity movement, training fasted is often fine. For longer sessions, higher intensity work or performance-focused training, fuelling beforehand can improve output, reduce stress load and support better adaptation. Training without fuel when intensity or duration demands it can increase fatigue, elevate stress hormones and compromise recovery. This is particularly relevant for women and for those already operating under high life stress.[57]

The question is not whether fasted cardio is 'good' or 'bad', it is whether it is appropriate for the session you are doing and the state your body is in.

Activity

Reflect on the following questions to see what opportunities exist when creating or optimising your exercise rhythm.

- In a typical week (not my best), how many times a week am I exercising?

(continued)

- What is my current exercise rhythm made up of (e.g., strength, zone 2 cardio, zone 5 cardio, balance and mobility work)?
- Am I currently missing any of the following types of exercise in my exercise rhythm: strength training, zone 2 cardio, zone 5 cardio/VO_2 max, balance and mobility work?
- What type of exercise do I want to focus on adding or being more consistent with when it comes to my exercise rhythm?
- What two to three types of exercise snacks feel easy for me to alternate and add into my day?

Conclusion

Diversifying your exercise portfolio to include cardiovascular training, resistance training and functional balance and mobility is one of the most important levers you have when it comes to protecting your future health.

Training in a way that improves both cardiovascular fitness and strength does more than help you feel better today. It boosts mood, energy and focus now, while paying dividends to your long-term physical function, independence and cognitive health.

And if this is a rhythm you struggle with, take the pressure off. Something is always better than nothing. Focus on consistency over intensity and build from there, and also sitting less!

Chapter Six

Stress and recovery—Building your stress capacity

We are living in an era of sustained, elevated stress—not occasional pressure, but ongoing load at low doses, and the data reflects it. In 2025, Headspace survey data showed that psychological distress increases sharply from early adolescence, peaking at around 65 per cent in 18- to 25-year-olds.[58] At the same time, nearly 59 per cent of Australian employees reported experiencing mental distress driven by work pressures such as workload, constant meetings and unrealistic expectations.[59]

Stress is no longer an exception in our lives, yet most of the advice on how to handle it has not evolved. It sounds generally something like avoid, reduce or eliminate stress from your life. That might sound all well and good in theory, but it does not necessarily translate in the real world.

This chapter is about learning how to meet, absorb and recover from stress in a way that fits your life. It is about building the capacity and resilience to handle your demands without burning out.

While we've been talking about energy as something you create through your behaviours and daily rhythms, how you recover plays a major role in how you show up tomorrow, next week, next month and in the years ahead. Your recovery rhythm shapes how much stress you can tolerate, how well you bounce back from it and how effectively you adapt over time.

Elite sport and the military understand this completely. They know recovery is not a luxury or an afterthought, but is paramount to performance and wellbeing as that is where the adaptation happens. Training stress is applied deliberately, and recovery is engineered just as deliberately. That is how athletes and operators get fitter, stronger and more resilient over time.

Most corporate environments expect sustained output with little recovery architecture. There's talk about resilience but rarely is it upskilled with the tools and capabilities to achieve it. Instead, recovery becomes something done reactively, only once the exhaustion, illness or burnout hits.

Proactive recovery is different. It is about building an intentional and proactive recovery rhythm into your life with varying cadences and behaviours that match on a day to day, week to week, year to year basis. When done like this, recovery not only returns you to a baseline level of operating, but it also elevates it.

So, to be clear, stress itself is not the enemy—unmanaged stress is. All stress really is, is a signal and, in the right dose, it is a powerful driver of adaptation. Your nervous system is built for contrast. Load and release, being on and being off—just like a car has an accelerator and a brake. The problem is that many of us are permanently switched on in a sympathetic state, driving with our foot on the accelerator and never touching the brake, or not switching into a parasympathetic rest and digest state. When you operate like this, you are never fully recovering and are gradually restricting your capacity over time.

Learning how to switch stress on and off is a skill. Building tolerance to stress is a capability, and like any capability, it can be trained. Establishing a predictable and intentional recovery rhythm is the end goal and a big part of how you build your capacity and stress tolerance.

If your goal is sustainability, while performing at a high level without slowly eroding your health, this is possible, but it does require the right rhythms to be in place. Having stamina and resilience is part of that, but capacity is something you build and train, and that is what this chapter is about.

Why proactive recovery is the missing link

Across elite sport and military settings, recovery is built directly into the performance architecture.

I have worked with seven professional sporting teams, Olympic medallists and consulted to Special Forces for the past six years. While these environments look different on the surface, the underlying principle is the same: stress is expected, load is planned and recovery is treated as the proactive, intentional, non-negotiable strategy that underpins it all.

In these elite environments, recovery is resourced, scheduled and protected. Training is periodised, with hard blocks followed by lighter ones. Many of today's top athletes openly credit their longevity to how seriously they take recovery, prioritising sleep, nutrition and structured recovery routines as much as the training itself. LeBron James, for example, is widely reported to invest heavily in sleep and a year-round recovery regimen to stay competitive into his late 30s. Novak Djokovic has repeatedly highlighted that his extended career is the result of rebuilding everything from nutrition and sleep to stress management and recovery habits, not just hitting more balls.[60]

The military operates in much the same way. Recovery is critical for maintaining decision quality, reaction time, emotional regulation and cognitive sharpness in high-stakes environments. Repeated operations that demand high physical and cognitive performance without adequate recovery do not build toughness, they create a liability, increasing errors, slowing reactions and undermining long-term readiness. During the Australian Special Forces selection course, for example, candidates experienced large drops in strength and power, and it took up to three weeks after the course for these measures to return to baseline, which highlights just how long full recovery from extreme combined stress can take.[61]

Now, contrast this with most corporate environments. In business, sustained output is expected without an equivalent investment in recovery. Long hours are praised and cognitive load is constant. The lines between work and home are blurred. Recovery, for the most part, is often something people attempt only once they are already depleted. Time off becomes a response to exhaustion rather than a proactive strategy for sustainable performance.

Before I present keynotes or workshops, largely to C-suite executives, senior leaders and high-growth founders, I run pre-session surveys to get a clear pulse check and tailor the session to the room. Regardless of the industry, role or level of experience, the same pattern appears. Most people I survey (consistently more than 75 per cent of each group) treat recovery as a luxury, or they feel guilty prioritising it. And, for the minority who try to prioritise it, very few see it for what it is: a performance accelerator and a competitive differentiator. While this surprises me, it also excites me that they have the opportunity for a huge gain (as do you reading this).

When you don't have a proactive recovery rhythm, you, by default, have a collapse plan. Your collapse plan might look something like, after you meet the deadline, win the deal, finish an important event, or the quarter closes, you get sick. Or it might look something like the reactive burnout holiday away, or the weekends spent catching up on sleep or lounging on the couch rather than doing activities with friends or your children.

Proactive recovery is different. It is intentional, structured and built by design around your life. This doesn't mean you won't feel fatigued, but you will have habits in place to help you bounce back. You will have regular moments where you have space to breathe and reset. This all starts by reframing your relationship with recovery, and when you do, everything becomes more sustainable, efficient and enjoyable. Green flags!

I know this because it is a mistake I made myself—the irony on this does not escape me. There I was, being paid to work with hundreds of the best athletes in the country, surrounded by excellence, helping ensure they were ready to perform at their peak, which largely included how they recovered, and yet I thought the same didn't apply to me?

I thought I could operate at one pace, flat out, always on, giving 150 per cent all the time. I told myself this was what made me better at my job, more productive, more committed and more resilient—remember, I thought 'I have more capacity than most'.

The reality could not have been further from the truth. I was operating on fumes and ignoring the early warning signs from my body and brain, brushing them off and 'pushing through'. But that did not make them go away, it only made them louder. What initially felt like fatigue or exhaustion turned into repeated bouts of sickness, and me sleeping through my alarm more than once—which I never do! In those moments, I'd rest for 'a day' telling myself I'd be better by then, rather than listening to my body and respecting the process. This cycle went on for years, which I am embarrassed to admit, and it's a little sad, looking back, that I put so much importance on so many other things and people, rather than myself.

I'd love to say I eventually got the memo and changed my ways, but the truth is, I only did when I was forced to stop, slow down and chase answers to why I was unwell for over 12 months with many days and weeks spent bedbound.

Stress is not the problem (our relationship with it is)

Stress needs a PR makeover, and it needs it fast. It has developed a serious reputation problem. When something feels important or threatening, your brain kicks off a built-in chain reaction that leads to your heart rate rising, your focus sharpening and your breathing speeding up. This is your body biologically preparing to act.

The issue most of us face today is that we are living in a state of chronic, low-grade activation. Not full fight or flight, but never fully at rest. Constant cognitive load, jam-packed diaries, traffic on the way to work, digital noise and blurred boundaries mean our nervous systems never receive a clear signal that it is safe to stand down. Over time, this chronic, low-grade stress adds to what researchers call *allostatic load*—the cumulative 'wear and tear' on the body and brain from repeated activation of the stress response.[62]

You experience that load across multiple domains, including physical, mental, emotional, social and sensory.

Before we look at the behaviours in your recovery rhythm, it would be good to do an audit to see how you might make some shifts and put more boundaries in place to help reduce your stress. Read the following list and see what speaks to you. This might include:

- switching off non-essential notifications on your phone and computer
- creating clear boundaries between work and home, around when you start and when you stop
- avoiding email and work messages on the weekend
- protecting your evenings from becoming a second workday
- being fully present with what you are doing; for example, when you are eating you are eating—not scrolling, not half-working, not half watching something else
- allowing for moments of silence and thoughts, rather than filling them with podcasts, phone calls or anything else.

This is where the idea of a 'third space' might be useful. Sociologist Ray Oldenburg described 'third places' as settings that are neither home nor work, where people gather, connect and feel a sense of community. In your day-to-day life, you can borrow this idea and use certain in-between spaces like a cafe stop, a walk, a gym session, even your commute as a kind of third space. Use these moments to be present, not to listen to a podcast or scroll on your phone, but to just be. Creating a buffer between the parts of your day where you are producing or performing and the parts where you are simply transitioning or resting.

At a biological level, that allows your body a chance to slow down, your stress hormones can start to fall and the 'rest and digest' branch of your nervous system can be re-engaged. Proactive intentional use of these small transition spaces can help reduce carry-over stress and contribute to building your capacity.

What doesn't kill you makes you stronger

Now you know stress is not the enemy, a far more helpful question becomes: 'If stress is unavoidable, how do I build the capacity to handle it well?'

I am so glad you asked! This is where a few key terms would be helpful for you to know.

Eustress

Eustress refers to beneficial or 'good' stress. This is the kind of stress that challenges you just enough to trigger adaptation, growth and resilience but not so much it causes damage or breakdown. It is exposure to the right kind of stress, at the right dose, that builds our capacity and stress tolerance, not its absence.

Biologically, this is how we all adapt. Take resistance training as an example. This 'trigger' makes muscles stronger, bones denser, the cardiovascular system more efficient and the nervous system more pressure tolerant. This idea sits at the heart of hormesis.

Hormesis

Hormesis is the principle behind this idea that small, controlled doses of stress stimulate growth, adaptation and resilience, while high doses cause damage, and too little stress leads to stagnation and decline. In simple terms, a little bit of stress followed by recovery makes you more capable, but too much stress or stress without recovery does the opposite. As we have evolved, our bodies have adapted to many such pressures including hunger, cold, heat, movement and periods of scarcity.

This is where understanding how to build your stress tolerance (or think of it as stress fitness) becomes a useful lens.

Stress fitness

I first heard this term used by Dr Paul Taylor in 2023 when we were both speaking at PwC's The Outside, and it immediately clicked. The idea of stress fitness captures something most people intuitively understand but rarely apply.

Like your physical fitness, your stress fitness is not fixed. It sits on a continuum. It can be built, and it can be lost.

If you avoid stress entirely, your tolerance drops. If you live in constant, unmanaged stress, it also drops. The goal is the right dose of challenge or exposure, followed by deliberate recovery.

This is why the fitness analogy works so well. We all understand that to improve our strength, we need to train consistently and progressively, and if we stop, we lose our strength capacity. Stress works the same way.

Using the principle of hormesis, short and controlled exposures to stress can actually build our capacity and resilience. Strength training, aerobic exercise, heat, cold, fasting and even cognitive challenge are examples of this.

When stress rises and falls, we adapt. When stress is constant, we overload ourselves. Our day-to-day lives are particularly good at undermining our stress fitness if we are not intentional, with constant low-grade cognitive and emotional stress.

Tip: You are built for challenge

Every system in your body — your muscles, bones, heart, brain — adapt to challenge by becoming stronger, more efficient and more capable. Demand paired with recovery is how capacity and resilience are built.

Building your stress tolerance

Your ability to build your capacity and resilience to tolerate stress comes from intentionally choosing to 'do hard things'.

One of the best examples of this is strength and cardiovascular training, which we explored in Chapter 5. While we already covered the benefits of exercise, so we won't go deep here, resistance training and cardio are deliberate forms of eustress. You apply load, you recover and you adapt.

When you choose manageable stress on purpose, your nervous system learns two skills:

1. How to switch on without panicking, and how to switch off without getting stuck there.
2. Over time, pressure feels more manageable, you handle pressure better and recovery happens faster.

This is where tools like heat and cold exposure fit. While I said on page xxii that you cannot ice bath your way out of sleep debt, which is true and something I stand by, what you can ice bath or cold shower your way out of, or at least improve, is your stress tolerance.

If the idea of an ice bath does absolutely nothing for you, I completely understand. I am in that camp too. But as we now know, doing hard things is good for us and key to building our capacity and stress tolerance.

Cold and heat exposure

The exposure to heat and cold creates real, measurable stress in the body. Cold drives a sharp nervous system response, raising heart rate and stress hormones, while heat loads the cardiovascular system in a way that looks like moderate exercise.

Unlike us, our ancestors did not have air-conditioning, central heating or Uber Eats for the nights they had no groceries and it was raining. They lived with heat, cold, wind, rain and seasonal change. Because of this, their nervous systems were trained by default to adapt to the elements. Much of this variation has been removed for us today by our creature comforts, so unless we intentionally design and expose ourselves to these conditions, it is easy to avoid them.

Before exploring cold and heat exposure further, it also needs to be said that these tools are not for everyone. If you have any underlying medical conditions, are pregnant or have concerns about your response to cold or heat, speak with your medical professional before experimenting with them in isolation or together in contrast therapy.

Cold exposure

Ice baths, cold showers, ocean swims in winter—oh my! These types of cold exposure trigger acute and chronic physiological responses in the body. Blood vessels in the skin constrict to reduce heat loss, and shivering increases heat production to help keep your core temperature stable. Heart rate rises, breathing becomes quick and shallow, and every instinct tells you to get out. This discomfort is the exact point of the exposure. If you can stay present, slow your breathing and show your nervous system that it can stay regulated under pressure, you are training your stress tolerance.[63]

Cold exposure also switches on the protective stress response in your cells and boosts brain chemicals like norepinephrine and dopamine, which are linked with feeling more alert, motivated and mentally clear. While I have dabbled with cold showers before, not very consistently if I am honest, I have started using cold exposure as a short reset in the middle of the day in recent months.

On the days I work from my office, which has both a sauna and ice bath, I do a contrast session after lunch a few days a week to support my afternoon focus. As a lion chronotype, this is when my energy and focus naturally dip. Between us, I do not love ice baths the way I love saunas, but I repeat to myself 'I can do hard things' while doing some breathwork and I definitely notice a clearer focus afterwards.

When practised progressively, cold exposure can build stress tolerance and is associated with improvements in perceived stress, sleep quality and aspects of wellbeing. A 2025 meta-analysis of cold-water immersion trials found benefits when exposure was brief, controlled and intentional (typically <15°C for at least 30 seconds), and it was linked with better sleep quality, lower self-reported stress and higher quality of life, with more mixed effects on mood.[64]

If this is something you are open to trying, and you have no medical contraindications, here is an evidence-aligned way to start:

- Begin with mild cold (around 10 to 15°C), which can be a cold shower.
- Keep exposure short at first, about 30 seconds to two minutes.
- Increase the time gradually as your tolerance improves.
- Avoid extremes or long immersions unless you have experience and supervision.

Heat exposure

The benefits of heat exposure are different to cold, but it follows the same core principle of controlled stress. Heat therapy places a steady, manageable load on the cardiovascular system, where your heart rate rises into a range experienced during moderate exercise, blood vessels widen to increase blood flow to the skin, and core body temperature rises by around one to two degrees.[65]

Research links regular sauna use, defined as around two to seven sessions per week for 15 to 20 minutes at 80 to 100°C, with meaningful improvements in cardiovascular health. These include lower blood pressure, reduced arterial stiffness, better blood vessel function, and a substantially lower risk of dying from cardiovascular disease. Repeated heat exposure trains the heart to handle load more efficiently by challenging it, allowing recovery and repeating that cycle over time.[66]

The benefits of heat exposure from sauna use include raising your core body temperature and heart rate, then, as you cool down, shifting into a more parasympathetic 'rest and digest' state with increased HRV.[67] This rise and fall in temperature, which can be created using a sauna, warm shower or bath, can amplify the natural evening drop in core body temperature. That drop in core body temperature is a key signal that supports sleep onset and deeper sleep, particularly when the heat exposure happens within two hours before sleep.[68] Repeated heat exposure also induces heat-shock proteins, which help protect and repair cells, and are thought to contribute to the cardiovascular and stress-resilience benefits seen with regular sauna use.[69]

If this is something you are open to trying, and you have no medical contraindications, here is an evidence-aligned way to start:

- Begin with milder heat, around 70 to 80°C in a sauna (or warm bath), for five to ten minutes.

- Keep sessions short at first and limit to two to three times a week.
- Increase gradually to 15 to 20 minutes at 80 to 100°C as your tolerance improves.
- Avoid extremes or sessions >20 minutes unless you're experienced and supervised; hydrate well (500 millilitres water or electrolytes before/after).

Contrast therapy

When heat and cold exposure are combined, it is often referred to as *contrast therapy* as it involves moving between short periods of heating and cooling, such as a sauna followed by brief cold exposure. This controlled contrast challenges circulation, temperature regulation and stress systems in deliberate ways. Protocols popularised through more recent work, including by Dr Susanna Soberg, often suggest accumulating roughly 11 minutes per week of deliberate cold exposure and around 57 minutes per week of heat (for example, in a sauna). These weekly accumulated timeframes should be spread across two to three sessions, and typically finish on cold so the body has to rewarm itself, potentially engaging brown fat and mild shivering.

Now you understand that not all stress is created equal, and that some forms of 'good stress', like resistance training, cardiovascular fitness, heat and cold exposure, are worth leaning into because they can help train your stress response. From here, we are going to go deeper into how to build your recovery rhythm, and the different behaviours and cadences you want your recovery rhythm to consist of over time.

Your recovery rhythm

I believe recovery is one of the most underutilised areas when it comes to wellbeing and performance outside of elite sport and military environments, which means it has huge potential! I see confusion around what recovery is, with common misconceptions being that it's a luxury or it's something you take when you need it. I also see it get associated with only a good night's sleep or some time on the couch watching your favourite series. While aspects of these can be forms of recovery, what I am referring to when I talk about your recovery rhythm is the behaviours and cadences that have been intentionally and proactively designed into your days, weeks, months and years to allow you to adapt to stress, build resilience and expand your capacity.

Recovery needs to be intentionally and strategically designed into the way you live and work. Now, this isn't about turning recovery into another full-time job, but it is about reframing your relationship with it; understanding how important it is to your health, wellbeing and performance; and finding a recovery rhythm that works for you.

Research on recovery rhythms shows that the most effective way to prevent burnout is not by relying on occasional long breaks, but by building short, regular moments of recovery into everyday life. Studies demonstrate that daily micro-recoveries create repeated parasympathetic resets, delivering the greatest cumulative gains in energy and performance. They are also the easiest to sustain inside high-demand routines or busy lives.[70]

You now understand that recovery is planned in elite sport, and it is built into operational rhythms in the military. The next step is to look at what type of recovery rhythms and habits you want to add into your life, proactively, over time.

Next, I take you through how you can start to think about recovery and help you start to build your recovery rhythm. This approach has largely been informed by how elite sports people structure their year. Most operate around one clear off-season, a handful of longer breaks often referred to as a bye, and then more frequent weekly and daily recovery strategies layered throughout the season.

For example, most winter sports like NRL and AFL teams follow very similar annual recovery rhythms (we touched on this on page 16). I know this well, having worked closely with both the GWS Giants and Cronulla Sharks for eight years each.

For these winter sports, their typical pre-season begins in November and runs through to late January or early February, when trial matches start. From there, teams transition into the in-season period, with games running from March through to August, followed by finals in September, if you make it.

During pre-season, players usually have two weeks away from structured training around Christmas and New Years. This is not a full switch off, but a period where they follow individualised programs at home. There is often a three- to four-day long weekend built in at some point as well.

Once teams move into trial matches and the competitive season, their weekly rhythm changes depending on when games are scheduled. Matches fall on different days and times each week such as Friday night, Saturday night or Sunday afternoon.

When a team has a shorter turnaround, for example, a six-day gap where they play on a Sunday and again the following Saturday, recovery becomes even more of a priority. When there is a longer turnaround, such as an eight-day gap, from a Saturday game to a Sunday game the following week, recovery is still essential, but training can afford to be more intense. Across this in-season phase, teams also have a couple of scheduled byes. These create deliberate opportunities for deeper recovery.

Outside of this, there is an emphasis on recovery every single day—from intentional practices after training to protocols around nutrition, supplements and sleep.

If you are reading this and thinking 'how does this apply to me?', I use this example to highlight how important recovery is for elite athletes who are not just pushing themselves physically but cognitively as well. While your days and weeks are likely more consistent than an athlete's in-season game schedule, what is often missing is intentional recovery in any meaningful format.

Like mine, most of our weeks operate on a seven-day cycle. That predictability makes it easier to anticipate what is coming and create our recovery rhythm. This is where daily recovery becomes the most powerful place for you to start.

A large 2022 systematic review of 22 studies found that short micro-breaks, usually under 10 minutes, consistently helped people feel more energised and less fatigued across the workday, with clear and reliable benefits for wellbeing.[71]

Like the nutrition chapter, I will step you through this in an intentional, sequential order to help you think about creating your recovery rhythm one layer at a time.

Daily recovery

Daily recovery is the foundation of your recovery rhythm. While sleep is a daily form of recovery, it has its own dedicated chapter, so for the purpose of this section, we are focusing on micro-breaks, which I like to call 'brain breaks', and how you can easily weave them into your day.

You will remember I spoke about ultradian rhythms back in Chapter 3. This gives you a helpful way to think about how to structure your day. It doesn't have to be an exact 90 minutes of work, 20 minutes of recovery, it can be at a rhythm that works for your day.

If a 20-minute brain break feels unrealistic for you, start with five minutes, or whatever fits your day. It is the consistency of these that matter the most. I typically encourage people to aim for three brain breaks across the day. It can be more if they are shorter, or fewer if your day only allows for that. Three brain breaks might look like one in the morning, one around lunchtime and one in the afternoon.

Brain breaks

Brain breaks are the term I use to describe the daily micro-breaks that are so important to your recovery rhythm. In essence, these are the moments you have across the day where you have intentional stimulant-free time that provides psychological detachment from your role or core tasks.

Chances are you may already have three breaks built into your day that look something like the following:

- a morning coffee break while scrolling social media and/or checking emails
- a lunch break that changes time depending on the day, and is often eaten at your desk
- an afternoon coffee or sugar hit, or sometimes both.

If these breaks already exist in your diary, brilliant! This means you're only upgrading what you do in these, and how you use them.

I also think I need to clarify that this is not an anti-coffee campaign—personally I *love* coffee, and it actually has a range of health and performance benefits, but in the context of what I am talking about here, coffee is a stimulant. We are looking at micro-breaks across the day that are intentional and stimulant-free.

So how might you switch up your day to include these brain breaks? Here's an example of what you might do on an office day and a home day:

Office day:

- Mid-morning: Five- to ten-minute walk around the block (where you pick a coffee up on your way back to the office)
- Lunch break: Allocated consistently in your diary, which you have outside on your own or you meet a friend. You keep your phone in your pocket or leave it back at the office
- Afternoon: Ten-minute walk around the block, followed by snack back at the office of Greek yoghurt, berries and nuts with a peppermint tea.

Home day:

- Mid-morning: Five- to ten-minute walk around the park close to your house (where you pick up a coffee on your way home)
- Lunch break: Allocated consistently in your diary, which you have on your balcony or verandah, and then go for a ten-minute walk once you have finished
- Afternoon: ten-minute meditation or NSDR (non-sleep deep rest) track, followed by two minutes of air squats and an afternoon snack plate with vegetable sticks, hummus, cheddar cheese and wholegrain crackers with a glass of water.

What has stayed the same? You're still having your three breaks per day. You're still having your coffee in the morning. You're still having lunch. You're still having something to eat and drink in the afternoon.

What has changed? You are being so much more intentional about what you are doing and when.

- Before your morning coffee, you're adding a short five-minute walk around the block before getting your coffee to allow movement, sunshine and an opportunity to downshift.
- Lunch you start to protect in your diary and commit to having it away from your desk. By either eating outside in the sunshine or meeting a friend, you are present in the moment and not distracted by your computer or your phone.
- When you start to get your afternoon dip around 3.30 pm, you go for a ten-minute walk around the block and then come back to the office to have your afternoon snack, which is high in protein, fibre and colours. This allows you time to decompress from the day and also nourish your body and brain for the afternoon.

This is just one example of how you can layer in intentional brain breaks across the day, but there are so many options you can choose from.

In essence, if it fits the criteria of being intentional, stimulant-free time, it's a brain break.

I have been taking brain breaks for the last five years, and I am a big believer in them. My favourite go-to is a short walk. I live in the city, so when I am working from home, I will usually head out for a quick loop near the harbour or through the botanical gardens. There are a few reasons I love this type of brain break: I get fresh air and time outside, the movement helps create energy and there is some pretty cool science behind being near green and blue spaces. Plus, nature is genuinely enjoyable to be around.

Research shows that spending time in green and blue spaces is associated with lower psychological distress and better overall mental health, including in urban settings like mine.[72] These environments also support relaxation by lowering stress-related markers such as cortisol and sympathetic arousal, and shifts toward brainwave patterns with increased alpha and theta activity, which are linked with mindfulness and a calmer, more restorative state.[73]

During seasons where I have long days or particularly cognitively taxing work, I deliberately step up my brain break game, as I know this is key to not only surviving the days and doing the work, but thriving and putting out the level of quality I want.

For example, while writing this book, alongside my usual go-to brain breaks, I added a few extras as my days were longer and more cognitively demanding than my normal schedule. On days I wrote at home, that included doing a puzzle or using a colouring-in book so I would stay off the social media scroll! When I was at the office, it might be a sauna and ice bath contrast session. And on the hot, 35-degree-plus days, I walked on the treadmill or did 20 minutes on the bike instead of heading outside.

Now, if you have gotten to the end of this section and you feel like 'Jess, I don't have 20 minutes', the main message here is to be intentional and take *some* stimulant-free time. If you can only spare a micro moment between calls, take that. If you can take a few minutes to make yourself a herbal tea and do two to three minutes of box breathing, do that. Again, something is better than nothing.

Overleaf are a few options for you to choose from based on the time you have available to you.

Three-minute options

These breaks are ideal between meetings or when you only have a few minutes.

- Walk around the office or up and down the stairs.
- Do two to three minutes of movement, such as air squats, sit-to-stands or star jumps.
- Complete two to three minutes of box breathing (see page 149).
- Do a mini stretch sequence.
- Walk to get yourself a glass of water or herbal tea.
- Take a two- to three-minute gaze break: step outside or to a window and let your eyes wander over the horizon or a distant view.

Less-than-one-minute options

Use these when you are between calls, emails or tasks.

- Stand up and move your body or shake it out: shake your hands, arms and legs for 20 to 30 seconds.
- Take three rounds of a physiological sigh (see page 149).
- Do a face release: unclench your jaw, soften your tongue from the roof of your mouth, relax your forehead and around the eyes.
- Look away from your screen and focus on something distant.

The key here is to be intentional, proactive and strategic. To start, I always suggest scheduling these in your diary. While we can all have the best intentions to do these things, it is also easy to get caught up on calls, emails, meetings or completing a project, and the next minute, half the day has evaporated. Using external reminders as circuit breakers helps bring back your awareness and helps set your day up for success with intentional, proactive brain breaks, which form the foundation of your recovery rhythm.

A word on breathwork with guest expert Kate Kendall

Kate Kendall is a leading Australian yoga teacher, author of Life in Flow, *and co-founder of Flow Athletic. She is known for translating breathwork, meditation and nervous system regulation into practical, accessible tools that help people slow down, recalibrate and reconnect.*

In our relentless (and often exhausting) pursuit of productivity and peak performance, we often overlook one of the most powerful tools we always carry with us: our breath.

The mystics and scientists across the times have seen it as both magical and methodical. It can be both practical and powerful and, above all, it's biological and drives much of what happens within us. It's gifted to us at birth and taken at death.

And one conscious breath is often all it takes to come back to the body from a place of stress and overwhelm.

Through my experience working with individuals striving for excellence on the field and in the office, I've seen the breath act as a reliable anchor. It offers a way to reduce anxiety and support a rhythm that honours productivity, performance edge *and* wellbeing. It reminds us that performance isn't just about output, it's about presence, intuition, instinct, adaptability and sustainable momentum.

In a culture that rewards speed and volume, conscious breathing invites us to slow down, not to lose pace but to sharpen it. Inhaling with intention and exhaling with release becomes a simple practice of resilience and clarity. It's from here that productivity becomes not only what we do, but how we operate: grounded, calm and fully engaged with the task at hand.

When we practice conscious breathing, we're not just inhaling oxygen. We're regulating our stress response, tuning our attention and inviting a sense of centred presence into whatever we're doing. For high performers, this matters. Sustainable performance is not about powering through exhaustion, but about repeatedly returning to a state where clear thinking and emotional regulation are possible. Breathwork provides a direct way to support this in real time.

Breath practices broadly fall into three categories: formal, informal and therapeutic.

Formal practice involves setting aside intentional time for a structured breathing practice, often with a specific purpose such as calming, downregulating, or energising the system.

Informal practice is where breath awareness is carried into everyday life. This involves noticing the breath more often and observing how it influences your state of mind. From this awareness, you can borrow simple elements from formal practice and apply them when needed. See 'low and slow' on page 149 as a starting point to come back to throughout your day.

Therapeutic experiences are typically facilitated one-to-one or in group settings, and may be referred to as breath journeys, rebirthing or conscious-connected breathing. These practices use more intentional, continuous breathing patterns to create shifts in the nervous system and access deeper emotional or somatic experiences. When held in a skilled, trauma-informed setting, they can support regulation, release and reconnection. However, they are not necessary for day-to-day recovery and are not the focus here.

For the purpose of your daily recovery rhythm, the goal of breathwork is regulation not intensity. This is why the techniques referenced throughout this section, such as box breathing, the physiological sigh and low and slow, are deliberately simple. They are designed to be used between meetings, before a call or during a short brain break to help settle the nervous system and restore focus in real time.

Three breathing techniques to restore in real time

Becoming aware of your breath throughout the day, particularly when you notice yourself feeling anxious or rushed, can be a powerful way to restore a sense of internal safety. Try the following techniques (also illustrated in figure 6.1, overleaf).

1. Box breathing

Focus on slowing down your breath. Once you are comfortable with the rhythm, breathe in for a count of three or four, hold at the top for same count, exhale for the same count and then hold for the same count. Repeat for a minute or two.

2. Physiological sigh

Inhale through the nose slowly. Pause briefly at the top. Without exhaling, sip in a little more air with another brief pause and then exhale through the mouth with a sigh or sound. Feel the shoulders drop, jaw soften and belly release. That's one round. Repeat twice more.

3. Low and slow

Breathing through the nose, allow the inhalations to effortlessly dig low and slow in the abdomen rather than shallow and chest-based, which is more closely associated with stress responses.

Other than eating and sleeping, breathing is the behaviour you repeat most often without thinking. When you begin to pay attention to it, it becomes one of the most powerful tools you have for changing how you feel, moment by moment, across the day.

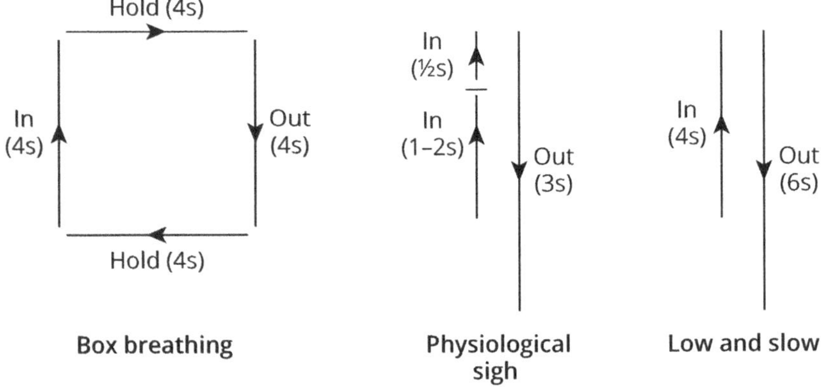

Figure 6.1 *Three breathing techniques for restoration*

Weekly recovery

Weekly recovery can start with you deliberately changing the pace of one day in your week. Similar to the daily forms of recovery, it can be from any number of behaviours. The purpose of this is to create contrast to your usual day-to-day activities of being on, performing and go-go-going.

Below is a list of ideas on how you might start to integrate a weekly recovery habit into your recovery rhythm:

- float tank session
- massage
- contrast therapy (sauna and ice bath)
- a few hours/half a day technology-free
- coastal walk

- half-day hike in nature
- yin yoga class
- family day with no schedule
- picnic in the park
- sound bath session
- breathwork session.

This is ultimately about creating contrast. If every day looks and feels the same, your nervous system never gets a clear signal to switch off. Regular psychological detachment from work and constant demands is linked to better recovery, lower stress and reduced risk of burnout. Even one intentionally different day each week, where rest, leisure or deeper recovery is protected, can interrupt the feeling that stress just rolls from one week into the next.

Over time, some of these weekly recovery habits may begin to happen more frequently, for example, the sauna may go from weekly to three or four times per week, like it has for me. The purpose of weekly recovery is to provide a deeper rest than daily brain breaks, but still at a regular cadence.

Quarterly resets

When I was working with various sports teams, including the Cronulla Sharks, GWS Giants AFL and AFLW, Western Sydney Wanderers, NSW Waratahs, Sydney Kings and Giants Netball, despite them being different codes with unique skills and training to match, they all had a few things in common.

One of those was a weekend off every few months. Typically, this would be once in pre-season, and also a couple of times when they were competing, in season. The purpose of this was to allow for a greater opportunity to physically and mentally freshen up.

Everyone can apply this same concept by adding in three quarterly resets each year. The fourth is replaced by an extended break, which for athletes is their off-season. Ideally, where possible, these quarterly breaks are roughly every three months so there is a consistent rhythm. You might be able to align these with many of the public holidays, but if not, I'd encourage you to think about taking a day off and creating these. Where possible, you want to try and get away, out of your normal routine, and away from the day-to-day activities.

What you choose is up to you. It might be time by the beach, in the country, a warm escape up north or a ski trip in the cooler months. All these work for the same reason: they take you out of your normal environment and away from constant cognitive demand.

Research suggests that it is not just 'time off' that matters, but getting out of your usual environment and mental groove. When you step away from your normal work settings and routine, it becomes easier to stop thinking about emails, deadlines and to-do lists, a process researchers call psychological detachment.[74] This kind of mental and physical change of scenery is consistently linked with better recovery, lower exhaustion, and improved mood and creativity.[75]

My favourite place to do this is the NSW North Coast, especially Byron Bay. Every time I go, I am struck by how quickly my physiology changes. My Oura ring and WHOOP band show this almost immediately. Better recovery scores, higher HRV, lower resting heart rate.

Research shows that even short breaks from work can meaningfully reduce stress and strain and improve wellbeing, with benefits lasting for weeks afterwards. The key here was getting outside of your usual environment.[76] So, if you've been thinking about booking a mountain cabin escape or a coastal weekend away, this might be your sign (and excuse) to do just that!

If it's not possible for you to take a long weekend away, think about how you can bring this concept to home. Can you be a tourist in your own city? Maybe you take an extra day off work, or you make the most of a long weekend when they land in the calendar. Maybe you do a day trip somewhere or take a ferry somewhere you haven't been before. An example for me is, I often get the ferry to Manly, but never to Watsons Bay. The key is making sure you are away from work, or anything that pulls you into that mode.

Annual recovery block

I am sure this one is not going to be a hard sell at all—the idea of taking one proper holiday each year for a complete reset. Think of it as your version of an athletes' off-season.

Potentially, the shift here for you might be reframing what this break is, or what it is made up of. I see a lot of people taking the burnout vacation, which I have had a few of before: crawling to the finish line, nervous system absolutely fried, and needing a complete reset just to get back to baseline.

The intention with these daily, weekly and quarterly recovery rhythms across the year is so you are getting to your big annual recovery time in a better state. Yes, fatigue will still be there, but this shift is you will be ready to take a break compared to feeling burnout.

Research has shown that people who have a holiday coming up often feel happier in the weeks beforehand than those who are not going away, likely because they are anticipating the break. But, only very relaxed holidays tend to boost happiness upon return, which is why the goal here is a 'holiday you don't need a holiday from'.[77]

I am sure you have had the feeling where your holiday is coming to an end, and you're thinking about when you can next book a break in the diary! This is your sign (or excuse) to do just that, even if it means just blocking your diary out for now.

Zoom out

Zooming out across the year means stepping back from your individual days and weeks and looking at the bigger picture. It is about understanding what your months and entire year look like.

To do this, you might print out your calendar to see what is ahead or look back at what your previous year looked like. If you don't want to do that, you can reflect on the following questions so you can identify what the rhythm of your year is typically like.

Reflection

Take a moment and look at last year and the year ahead, and answer the following questions:

- When are your busiest periods with work?
- When are your quieter periods with work?
- When does life outside of work demand more of you?
- Is there a time of year (or times) where you typically get rundown or sick?

When you can zoom out and start to understand what the rhythms of your year look like, you can embed a proactive annual recovery rhythm. It is not waiting until you are exhausted and then booking leave, it is looking back, noticing patterns and planning.

I will be honest; this went out the window for me last year. It was my first year navigating motherhood while also running a business.

There was lot of surviving and figuring things out as I went, and not as much rhythm as I would have liked. On a daily and weekly level, my resets were pretty good, but the quarterly resets and annual recovery block were non-existent.

This year, I want to do better, and I know it starts with taking the time now to map out my year with intention. Your yearly rhythm needs to include work and home life.

Use your calendar to support this. This doesn't mean every detail must be locked in (unless that's how you like to operate). Life moves and things shift, but having visibility gives you structure and will help you implement your annual recovery rhythm. You are also far more likely to follow through when you set this up while you are fresh, rather than already depleted.

Case study: Finding your yearly recovery rhythm

Gabrielle, a CEO and mother of three young children, came to me as she was tired, getting sick often and would spend her weekends on the couch recovering rather than filled with the energy she wanted for activities with her family. She knew something needed to change.

During our coaching, we first worked on her nutrition, exercise and sleep rhythms. We then moved to her recovery rhythm, starting with a few brain breaks, which included a nourishing snack, a lunchtime gym session and a walk around the block in the afternoon. Then we moved on to weekly forms of recovery, and she started having a sauna one to two times per week and also taking some time on the weekend to go for a walk.

(continued)

She was already doing a pretty good job of the quarterly breaks by default. She would schedule time off work to spend with her children, and they would go away camping, to visit family or overseas.

Where she really found value was when we started discussing what her year looks like. I remember, at the start, she said there were periods where she would often have to work when she got home. So, we mapped them out. She also got clear on when school holidays, her industry's peak periods and the workload for a new course she was studying would occur.

She could suddenly see the rhythm of her whole year, and visibility gave her back control. Around that, she made sure she had scheduled her quarterly resets, and we discussed how, for her, it was the daily and weekly recovery practices that were going to be very important.

This visibility of the year from a work and life perspective helped give her clarity on when she may have to say 'no' to things, to prioritise herself, her recovery and her energy.

This is the difference between sustaining energy and constantly playing catch-up. It is the difference between living proactively and living reactively. And I know how both feel. I much prefer living in alignment with a rhythm. For me, this year's plan has been to take a long weekend each month. Fridays are days I spend with my daughter, but last year, I would find myself squeezing something in: a meeting, a deadline, a bunch of emails. So, this year, I am focusing on being intentional and present, and that starts with boundaries—which means not agreeing to any calls or anything extra on a Friday and just politely saying 'sorry I am not available'.

For that 'long weekend', I try to do something different to change up my routine, such as going to a different cafe or beach or taking a new route on a walk. Basically, I am trying to get out of default mode, change things up and be a tourist in my own city.

Tip: Mindful planning for recovery

Your year will look and feel completely different when you know what's coming and give yourself moments for intentional recovery pauses.

Activity

Before you begin, remember this - your wellbeing and leading a sustainable high-performance life is built on intentional, strategic recovery, not constant output. This activity is here to help you shift from waiting until you are exhausted to recovering with intention, so you can protect your energy, sharpen your thinking and build the capacity required for the long run.

Now it's time to design your annual recovery rhythm, and the best place for you to start is with your daily recovery — your brain breaks.

1. Are you currently taking any brain breaks across the day?
2. From the brain breaks examples in this chapter, identify three options that feel realistic, enjoyable and easy to integrate into your day. If you work from the office and home, write a list for both.
3. What needs to be in place to make these happen consistently (for example, scheduling them in your diary and setting reminders)?

(continued)

Now, go and schedule brain breaks into your diary for the duration that works for your schedule.

Once your brain breaks become a regular part of your day, move on to planning your weekly, quarterly and annual breaks.

This may take you weeks or months to execute, which is fine. Don't rush. You want to leverage the energy and momentum each part of your annual recovery rhythm creates.

Conclusion

Ultimately, your annual recovery rhythm is designed to deliberately create space to downshift and recover from the pressure of day-to-day life. These intentional moments do more than just bring you back to baseline. They allow you to adapt, rebuild and expand your capacity over time, ultimately elevating the energy you have and how you move through your days, weeks and years.

Most of what I have outlined in this chapter is genuinely enjoyable. Ice baths might be the exception, but even there, the value lies in choosing challenge on purpose and becoming comfortable doing hard things. As the saying goes: 'Hard choices, easy life. Easy choices, hard life.'

Now you understand the different behaviours and cadences that can make up your annual recovery rhythm, the next step is to start applying them. This means thoughtfully considering how this rhythm fits into your life, and where small intentional changes make the most sense.

As mentioned earlier, this section has been designed to be followed sequentially. My recommendation to you is to start by focusing on what you can do on a daily basis, your brain breaks, as these will deliver you the biggest impact to your day and life.

Chapter Seven

Sleep—The ultimate recovery

You might have heard the saying, 'win the morning, win the day' with respect to how important morning routines are. And, I agree, how you start your day matters. But to really win the day, you need to win the night first.

Sleep is the most important form of recovery we have, given we spend one-third of our life doing it, and it is anything but passive. There is so much happening when you sleep! This is when your brain clears waste, your body repairs tissue, your emotions are processed and your memories are transferred from temporary to permanent storage. Sleep is also where your immune system manufactures your immune fighting cells. Of all the recovery tools available to us, sleep is the most powerful. And, yet, it is the one many of us struggle with.

More than half of adult Australians experience at least one chronic sleep symptom that interferes with daily functioning.[78] Almost 60 per cent regularly struggle with issues such as difficulty falling asleep or staying asleep, and close to 15 per cent report symptoms consistent with clinical insomnia. Sleep is widely valued, yet increasingly difficult to achieve.

Part of the challenge is that many people find it hard to switch off, especially if your days are high-octane with back-to-back meetings, constant decision-making, travel and stress. This way of operating has your foot to the floor all day. It's like pulling into your driveway after a long drive on the freeway. You don't pull into the driveway at the same speed you are on the freeway; you slow down. If you drive a manual, you downshift through the gears.

How many people operate on a daily basis is the same as pulling into their driveway at top speed. They are operating at full pace right up until bedtime, and expect their body to instantly power down. Sleep does not work like that.

That is often why thoughts feel busy when you get into bed, or why you fall asleep initially, only to wake in the middle of the night with your mind alert and active, which leaves us feeling tired but wired.

My relationship with sleep has not been uncomplicated. As a teenager, I experienced sleep anxiety. In my mid-20s, sleep was disrupted again, this time by anxiety and panic attacks following a traumatic incident that resulted in PTSD and insomnia for a period of time. And now, as a new mum, I am navigating an entirely different set of sleep challenges. Fellow parents—IYKYK!

Despite all of this, I am a self-proclaimed sleep enthusiast. I genuinely love sleep! I love getting into bed with clean sheets. I love waking after an uninterrupted night feeling clear, rested and ready to go. I am even that person who travels with their own pillow. You get the point, sleep *really* matters to me.

My appreciation of sleep has not come easily or by accident. Couple that with me seeing just how interconnected sleep is with nutrition, recovery and nervous system health, it is crystal clear that sleep really is the bedrock of health and performance, and it needs to be prioritised like anything else of significance in your life.

What's the saying? We make time for what matters. Think about anything that is truly important to you. It lives in your calendar so you do not forget it. That is exactly how sleep needs to be treated. Not as something you fit in if the day allows, but as a non-negotiable appointment. One you keep every single night, and you don't skip, cut corners on or neglect.

The point I want to leave you with is this: if sleep feels hard or you constantly feel tired and wired, you are not alone, and the great news is that there's likely a lot within your control. And, while there are genuine medical sleep conditions that require professional assessment and treatment, most everyday sleep disruption sits within the realm of habits, rhythms and recovery rather than pathology.

This means sleep is often able to be influenced far more than you might think. In the following sections, we will focus on building the conditions that allow sleep to do what it is designed to do: help us feel rested, restored and energised!

Why sleep has become so challenging

What shapes sleep more: nature or nurture?

As we've explored in Chapter 3 with your circadian rhythm, your biological wiring has not changed for thousands of years, but the environment has. Artificial light extends the day, work bleeds into evenings, and meals, movement and rest shift later or become inconsistent. All of which result in it being harder for us to either get to sleep or stay asleep.

The reality is, a good night's sleep starts long before your head hits the pillow. When things like meals, movement, light exposure and rest happen with some consistency, the transition into sleep is easier. But, when those cues are inconsistent or pushed later, the body struggles to slow down and prepare to sleep, making sleep more challenging for many of us.

Common disruptors to sleep include:

- difficulty switching off
- chronic stress
- screens and late-light exposure
- flexible work and blurred boundaries
- late exercise and late eating
- caffeine
- alcohol
- sleep anxiety and performance pressure around 'getting enough' sleep
- revenge bedtime scrolling.

Getting a good night's sleep now requires us to intentionally set boundaries and behaviours—and it is happening at a time where our energy, attention and capacity are already stretched. You can see the mismatch happening!

Your sleep architecture

Remember how we spoke about ultradian rhythms back in Chapter 3? Well, your sleep cycle is a great example of this in action. Sleep runs in repeating cycles across the night, and each cycle contains different stages that are unevenly distributed, and they do not all serve the same purpose. Your sleep cycles broadly follow the following patterns.

Stage 1: Transition

This is the lightest stage of sleep and the bridge between wakefulness and sleep. Brain activity shifts from relaxed awake (alpha) towards theta, muscles relax, and your heart rate and breathing begin to slow. You can still wake easily here.

Stage 2: Light

Here, the body starts to properly settle. Body temperature drops, breathing and heart rate slow, and muscle tone decreases. The brain becomes less responsive to outside noise and movement. We spend the largest proportion of the night, typically around 45 to 55 per cent of total sleep, in this state.

Stage 3: Deep sleep

This is also referred to as slow-wave sleep, and in this stage, your brain produces delta waves. This is the most physically restorative stage of sleep, where growth hormone is released and tissues are repaired. In this stage, the glymphatic system clears metabolic waste from the brain. You get more deep sleep in the first half of the night, which is one of the reasons consistent bedtime matters. You typically spend about 15 to 25 per cent of the night in deep sleep.

Stage 4: REM sleep (a separate stage that sits alongside the three NREM stages)

In rapid eye movement (REM) sleep, brain activity becomes highly active and looks more like wakefulness. This stage supports memory consolidation, learning, emotional processing and creativity. Here, dreams are move vivid, and muscles are paralysed to prevent you acting them out. REM periods become longer and more dominant in the second half of the night. You usually spend 20 to 25 per cent of the night in REM sleep.

Across a typical night, you move through four to six of these cycles, each lasting around 90 minutes, with earlier cycles having more deep sleep and later cycles having more REM sleep.

You can see why, when it comes to sleep, there's a lot more to consider than just time in bed. There's time you actually slept, how restorative that sleep was, and so on, so it really is about *quantity* and *quality*.

There are different stages or phases in life where sleep can become particularly difficult—my fellow parents, you know what I am talking about! I know, for myself, right now, to get my preferred seven to eight hours of sleep, I need to spend more time in bed than usual as I am often woken a few times a night (on a good night!). Because I use a wearable device, I was able to figure out that, on average, for me to get 7.5 hours of sleep, I need to be spending between eight to nine hours in bed.

Where wearables have a place

In my opinion, this is also where sleep tracking devices can be useful. Wearables (which we covered in Chapter 2) are best at showing patterns over time. They help you see how factors like travel, stress, alcohol or late meals impact your sleep.

Their real value is not in the accuracy of any single night, but the consistency of the data when the same device is worn regularly. When paired with how you feel subjectively, this data can provide useful feedback and a more complete picture of what is really happening—like it did for me in Queenstown!

Used well, wearables are a reflection tool. They are most helpful when they prompt curiosity rather than judgement, and when they support awareness rather than obsession.

Tip: Health benefits of sleep

During deep sleep, your brain switches into clean-up mode.

A network called the glymphatic system clears out the metabolic waste that builds up across the day. One of the key substances removed is beta-amyloid, a protein that has been linked to Alzheimer's disease when it accumulates over time.

Setting yourself up for sleep success

It's important to understand that sleep starts long before your head hits the pillow. It begins the moment you wake up. How you structure your day determines how easily you fall asleep, how deeply you stay asleep and how restored you feel the next morning.

Foundations before fixes

Before supplements, gadgets or optimisation strategies, sleep needs a consistent foundation. Cognitive demand, stress, meal timing, light exposure and the absence of micro-breaks accumulate across the day, impacting how you get to sleep or stay asleep at night. Being aware of this, as well as looking at some of the key environmental and timing factors, will help set you up with a strong sleep rhythm.

Work with your biological timing

As we covered in Chapter 3, your circadian rhythm is heavily influenced by light exposure. Morning daylight on the eyes is one of the strongest signals for setting the sleep-wake cycle, helping anchor energy earlier in the day and melatonin release later at night.

Your sleep chronotype (which we also covered in Chapter 3) is another factor that plays a role. Knowing whether you are a lion, bear, wolf or dolphin helps you understand your natural sleep-wake preference and when your energy and focus are likely to peak. Wherever possible, align your sleep/wake times and your most cognitively demanding work with this biological rhythm rather than push against it.

Create a sleep sanctuary

Sleep quality is highly sensitive to environment. Your body sleeps best when the bedroom is cool, dark and quiet. Here's how you can achieve this:

Stay cool

A cooler room supports the natural drop in core body temperature of around 1 to 2°C that accompanies falling asleep. Most adults sleep best in a cool room, often around 16 to 20°C, with some individual variation.

You can set the thermostat or use a fan, pre-cool the room 30 minutes before bed, or use a warm shower or sauna one to two hours earlier. The heat triggers vasodilation, followed by an after-drop in body temperature that supports sleep onset.

Consider the lighting

Darkness supports your natural melatonin rhythm. Evening light, especially bright or blue-rich light, can suppress or delay melatonin production. Use blackout curtains or an eye mask, remove light sources such as charging docks and clocks, dim lights in the evening, and avoid screens in the hour before bed as much as possible.

Keep it down

Noise fragments sleep, even when you do not fully wake, by causing brief arousals and shifts into lighter sleep. Earplugs or white noise can reduce arousal thresholds and reduce these micro-arousals in noisy environments. I, personally, use both a white noise machine (I am all about the rain noises) and the QuietOn 4 noise-cancelling sleep earbuds.

The way you want to think about your bedroom is as a behavioural cue signalling that this room is for two things: sleep and intimacy. It's not your cinema or your restaurant or your doom scrolling place. When you are strict about this, it helps with the cognitive and behavioural cues that help your brain wind down for sleep.

Sleep loves consistency

There's my favourite word again! Sleep works best when timing is predictable. Regular sleep and wake times strengthen your circadian rhythm and reduce the effort required to fall asleep. When wake and sleep times are most consistent, your sleep onset becomes easier and your overall sleep architecture tends to improve. When your schedule is consistent, your brain learns the pattern, sleep onset becomes easier and your sleep architecture, especially your deep and REM cycles, tend to improve over time.[79]

Variable bedtimes disrupt circadian signalling and are linked with greater day-to-day sleepiness and higher cardiometabolic and psychological risk, even when total sleep time looks okay on paper. Research shows that more regular sleep timing is associated with better health, including cardiometabolic outcomes, improved mental health and often better daytime functioning and alertness, compared with irregular sleep schedules.[80]

There are practical steps you can take to improve your sleep quality.

Set fixed anchors

Choose your wake time first (aim for within about 30 minutes each day, including on weekends) and then aim for a bedtime that gives you enough opportunity to sleep.

Shift gradually

If you are trying to align your sleep times with a schedule that better suits your needs, use incremental 15-minute shifts toward your target. Morning light exposure and consistent eating times can work as cues to signal your body it's time to wake up and help anchor your rhythm earlier in the day.

Track your schedule

This process is not a set and forget. Play with your sleep and wake times for two weeks to find your sweet spot. Aim for 80 to 85 per cent schedule adherence before tweaking the duration.

Eat earlier, not later

As outlined in Chapter 4, *what* you eat and *when* you eat both matter. Spreading your intake out to be more evenly distributed across the day, and allowing a few hours between your last meal and bedtime, is often associated with better metabolic outcomes and, in many studies, better sleep quality. This sits within the field of chrono nutrition, which looks at how the timing of food interacts with your circadian rhythm to influence energy, metabolism and sleep.[81]

Large, late meals increase digestive and metabolic activity at a time when the body should be winding down. WHOOP has found that members who eat closer to bedtime are associated with 26 minutes of less sleep, 3 per cent less REM sleep and a 10 per cent drop in next-day recovery scores.[82]

Eating earlier supports night-time recovery by reducing the demand on your digestion during sleep. This helps align your eating rhythm with your biology for a better night's sleep.

Train with sleep in mind

Exercise is one of the most powerful tools for improving sleep quality, but timing and intensity matter. A recent large-scale data analysis study from Monash University, analysing almost 15 000 active adults and over four million nights of sleep, showed that strenuous evening exercise ending within four hours of bedtime was associated with delayed sleep onset, shorter sleep duration, lower sleep quality, higher resting heart rate and lower HRV overnight. When exercise finished more than four hours before sleep, these disruptions were no longer seen.[83] Earlier movement, particularly at lighter to moderate intensity, consistently supported better sleep quality.

This does not mean evening training is off-limits. It means, where possible, be intentional with your exercise rhythm. Running, HIIT and team sports are stimulating by nature, so if they sit later in the day, build in extra downshifting time or habits, or ideally keep later sessions lighter.

Cue your landing

Evening routines do not need to be elaborate. Their role is to signal to your body and brain that it is time to shift from doing to recovery.

The next section brings these foundations together into a practical sleep landing protocol designed to be something you can adapt and, most importantly, do consistently.

Your sleep landing protocol

Sleep works best when it is approached intentionally and consistently.

The way I like to think about how you should prepare to sleep each night is the same as a plane preparing to land. A plane does not drop out of the sky and hit the runway (thank goodness!). Every landing follows a structured process, where the same sequence of events happens. You're asked to put your big electronics away and your tray tables up. Then it's small electronics off and seatbelts on. The cabin crew take a seat for the final part of the descent.

It doesn't matter where the plane is flying to or who is in the cockpit. This part of the trip is standardised across every aircraft, and if you're a frequent flyer, you can probably recite the script. Sleep works the same way, or at least it should.

Having a sleep landing protocol becomes a game-changer. When I talk about a sleep landing protocol, it has two parts: the descent and the touchdown.

Part one: The descent

Just like every flight follows the same sequence of events for each descent, this part can be standardised for all of us. These are research-backed steps that you can implement across your day to set your night up for sleeping success.

Cut caffeine

Caffeine has a relatively long half-life of about four to six hours (sometimes longer), so it can still be circulating in your system ten to 12 hours later. Research suggests that a typical cup of coffee (around 100 mg of caffeine) should be consumed at least nine hours before bedtime to avoid measurable reductions in total sleep time. To set yourself up for sleep success, aim to cut your caffeine intake nine hours before you go to bed, especially if you struggle with sleep onset or depth.[84]

Adjust food timing

Large meals close to bedtime increase metabolic and digestive activity at a time when your body should be winding down. Leaving around three hours between your last substantial meal and bed can make it easier to fall asleep and may support more restorative sleep, especially if you tend to eat late or experience night-time wakings. If you get hungry, you're better off having a smaller high-protein snack closer to bed and keep dinner earlier where possible.

Remove stimulation

About an hour before bed, start winding things down. That means stepping away from screens and anything that fires up your brain. This is partly about light exposure, but even more about mental activation. Engaging content keeps your brain in 'on' mode for longer than you realise, increasing cognitive and emotional arousal and making it harder to switch off and get to sleep. In simple terms, if your mind is still switched on, sleep must wait.

For me, I am strict on numbers 1 and 3: I am very caffeine sensitive, and the same for screens and what I am consuming. There is a constant debate at my house on what we will watch at night. I really don't like to consume anything too suspenseful as I know it takes me longer to wind down—no, I don't want to watch a crime documentary right before I go to bed, and, yes, I'd much prefer *Real Housewives* or *Below Deck*, which allows me to switch off more (yes, I love some trashy TV). Dinner is the one I struggle with, especially in this season of life with a one-year-old, but I do the best I can, which is also the same point I want to make to you—do the best you can.

Part two: The individualised touchdown

Like each flight, this part is personalised to you. This is about you choosing an easy and repeatable sequence of habits you do each night, so your body and brain can recognise the pattern and cognitive cuing that are setting you up for sleep success. The goal is to create something simple, repeatable, with one clear message to your brain—we are preparing to land!

The goal is a calm, consistent, predictable touchdown each night. To start, choose two or three small, repeatable behaviours that signal to your body and brain that you are starting to switch from *doing* to *recovery* mode as you prepare to land for the day. This might include things like:

- taking a hot shower or bath
- brushing your teeth
- cooling the bedroom
- having a magnesium drink (bisglycinate or threonate)
- sipping a relaxing herbal tea
- reading (preferably a hard copy book or an e-reader, which has much less blue light emission than a phone or tablet). Also try not to read something too engaging—for me this is not the time for personal or professional development, I keep those books for the morning or daytime!
- journalling
- writing tomorrow's to-do list
- reflecting on three wins from your day and three wins for tomorrow
- listening to a meditation track
- breathwork.

There is not some magical formula that is superior to the rest, it is about what works for you, and what you can do consistently!

Remember, the main purpose of this is to trigger a consistent cue to your brain. When we do these things, we get ready to sleep.

You may find you have your standard landing protocol but, at times of high stress, you may need to dial these strategies up and add an extra one or two in. But, don't start with extra steps, we are all about the path of least resistance here.

For example, my individualised touchdown (at the moment) is:

- magnesium drink
- hot shower
- skin routine
- one of the following: listen to a sleep meditation track, or journal in my diary about three wins from the day and three wins for tomorrow. (I got this from one of my favourite books, *The Gap and the Gain* by Dan Sullivan and Benjamin Hardy.)

When I am feeling a bit more stressed than usual, which generally shows up as me struggling to get to sleep, I dial the routine up a bit more and generally do all of the above. I might even refrain from watching any TV in the evening and replace it with reading a book, doing a puzzle or having a sauna if I haven't already had one.

Naps, Nappucinos and NSDR

If you struggle to get enough sleep at night, there are a few strategies you can use across the day to help close the gap and support your recovery. The key is choosing what works for you.

Naps

To nap or not to nap—that is the question. Naps tend to divide people: some people love them, others avoid them at all costs as they know they will pay for it later. Naps are not inherently good or bad. Whether they help or hinder your sleep depends on how, when and why you use them.

If you are going to nap, two factors matter most.

1. Timing

Early afternoon is the safest window for a nap, when your circadian rhythm naturally dips one or two hours after lunch. Napping too late in the day increases the risk of cutting into your sleep drive and making it harder to fall asleep at night, especially if combined with the next factor.

2. Duration

Short naps are generally better tolerated than long ones. A brief nap of 20 minutes or less is ideal so you don't go into deeper stages of sleep, which will limit grogginess when you wake. Longer naps increase the likelihood of sleep inertia and can interfere with night-time sleep, particularly if you are already struggling with sleep quality.[85]

Nappuccinos

Research on a caffeine-nap, also referred to as 'nappuccinos', has gained some attention. This strategy involves consuming caffeine immediately before a short nap, because caffeine takes around 20 to 30 minutes to exert its stimulating effects. The idea is that you wake as the caffeine begins to work, combining the restorative effect of a nap with improved alertness. For some people, this can be effective. For others, particularly those sensitive to caffeine or prone to sleep anxiety, it can backfire and increase evening restlessness. As with most sleep strategies, your individual response and preference matters.[86]

Personally, I am not a good napper. If I nap, I almost always regret it. It impacts my ability to fall asleep later and disrupts my sleep rhythm. I only know this because I have paid attention to what happens after a nap. Almost every time, I struggle to fall asleep that night and lie there regretting the decision. Because naps don't work for me, I have experimented with other techniques, including non-sleep deep rest (NSDR). I find it far more restorative in the moment without compromising my sleep later that night.

Non-sleep deep rest (NSDR)

NSDR is an umbrella term for practices such as Yoga Nidra and guided, body-based relaxation, where you say awake but enter a deeply relaxed state. These sessions are designed to downshift the nervous system—breathing slows, muscle tension drops and physiological markers of stress tend to decrease—without actually falling asleep. Some of the shifts include brain activity toward more relaxed patterns and reduced autonomic arousal, helping you take your foot off the accelerator.

NSDR works particularly well as a daytime reset or brain break. A short, structured relaxation session can reduce perceived stress and mental fatigue and improve subsequent focus, without the sleep inertia or night-time disruption that some of us experience with naps. Curious to give it a try? You can search 'NSDR track' on Spotify or YouTube until you find one you like based on voice, style and length. I often use Mindset Change or Dr Andrew Huberman NSDR tracks, and I just pick the duration that matches the time I have available.

Set an alarm, just not the one you think!

Most people think the solution to better mornings is a different wake-up alarm. It's not. For the next two weeks, I want you to experiment with a go-to-bed alarm.

To do this, pick your ideal wake time, then count backwards eight to nine hours to find your target bedtime. Now set an alarm for 45 to 60 minutes before that time. When it goes off, that's your cue to close the laptop, pause the show, put your phone on charge outside the bedroom and start part 2 of your sleep landing protocol.

You can expect your future self to bargain with you—'just one more email' or 'just one more episode' or 'I just need to finish this episode' or a final doom scroll temptation. The alarm is there is bring you out of these temptations and act as an external circuit breaker and cue saying, 'It's time to start getting ready to go to bed'.

This is particularly useful if you are trying to reset your sleep and wake times.

Case study: Redesigning sleep patterns

Ana wanted to start waking earlier. At the time, she was waking around 7 am and already felt behind before the day had properly started. Her goal was to wake at 6 am.

She had been trying to do this the way most people do. By setting an earlier wake-up alarm. But every time her alarm went off, she hit snooze, and she still got out of bed closer to 7 am.

So, we flipped the approach. Instead of only focusing on the morning, we started with the night before. We set a go-to-bed alarm for 9.15 pm. This was her cue to begin her wind-down routine. Her wake-up alarm was set for 6.45 am, only 15 minutes earlier.

Her wind-down routine ended up being a magnesium drink, a hot shower, washing her face and brushing her teeth, and then reading a few pages of her book in bed.

As her bedtime became more consistent, falling asleep became easier, her sleep quality improved and she started waking just before her alarm. We tracked this both through how she felt during the day and objectively using her Oura ring.

Over the following months, we gradually moved her wake time earlier in 15-minute increments. First to 6.30 am. Then 6.15 am. And eventually 6 am. Each shift happened only once her body was naturally waking just before the alarm.

Ana told me this was one of the easiest shifts she had made. She also mentioned that the hot shower at night allowed her to decompress and run over things from the day, which she was previously doing when she got into bed. Green flags!

Common sleep issues

How does getting a better night's sleep sound to you? Two of the biggest issues most of us face is difficulty falling to sleep or waking in the middle of the night and struggling to fall back to sleep. Here's a look at what might be happening, and most importantly, what you can do about it.

Difficulty falling asleep

Difficulty falling asleep is one of the most common sleep complaints, especially if you're carrying a heavy mental load.

It can often feel like you're physically tired and ready to sleep, but you're mentally wired, with thoughts racing as soon as your head hits the pillow, and the more frustrated you get about being awake, the harder it becomes to switch off. The catch 22 is the stress then drives your inability to sleep. Classic!

Heightened cognitive arousal, from thinking, planning and worrying, is one of the strongest predictors of trouble falling asleep. This situation is commonly fuelled by days that are back-to-back and go-go-go. It might look like full workdays with minimal breaks (no intentional brain breaks), rushing in traffic or between pickups, and that extra afternoon coffee that felt helpful at 4 pm, but not at 10 pm when you can't sleep.

Tip: Set yourself up for sleep success

- Build in three intentional brain breaks across your day.
- Implement the two stages of the sleep landing protocol (see page 170).
- Create and protect your sleep sanctuary. Remove clocks if you clock watch and don't bring your phone into your room.

Waking during the night

If you fall asleep without much trouble but often wake between 1 and 4 am with your mind in overdrive, you're not alone. Many people in high-responsibility roles describe lying awake and replaying conversations, running through to-do lists or mentally planning the day ahead.

This pattern is often about mental load: high decision-making demands, and ongoing cognitive or emotional strain keep your brain in a low-level alert state. At night when external distractions drop away and your mind finally has space to process, it switches into problem-solving mode right when you'd rather be asleep.

Here are a few things you can do before bed to reduce the risk of this happening, and if it still does, a few strategies you can turn to at night.

Before bed:

- Do a brain dump before bed: spend a few minutes writing out whatever is on your mind. It might be work related, life related or both. It might be worries, to-dos or anything unfinished.
- Create and implement your sleep landing protocol.

What to do if you wake up:

- Reframe unhelpful thinking. If you get stuck on the 'I must get back to sleep' script, try and reframe this and remind yourself that resting is still restorative and brief wakings are normal. This helps lower the pressure that is building.
- Give your brain a neutral anchor. Use something simple and repetitive like slow breathing (box breathing from page 149), a gentle body scan or counting breaths to help keep your attention away from planning and worry.
- Use the 20-minute rule. If you're clearly awake and not getting drowsy, get out of bed, keep the lights low and do something quiet and boring that does not involve your phone or bright screens until sleepiness returns, then go back to bed.

Case study: The 15-minute thinking block

I regularly work with senior leaders, C-suite executives and entrepreneurs. These are the people most likely to wake in the middle of the night with a busy mind, particularly when their operating system lacks enough opportunities to properly charge down.

After delivering a sleep session to a group of senior executives, a senior Australian businesswoman shared what became a game-changer for her. She began scheduling a dedicated 15-minute thinking block first thing in the morning.

Previously, she would wake overnight with thoughts about the day ahead and feel the need to mentally work through them in the moment. By pre-allocating time in the morning to address those thoughts, she no longer felt pressure to solve them at 3 am. If she woke during the night, she could reassure herself that there was a set time to deal with everything the next morning, which made it far easier to settle back into sleep.

Medical sleep issues

You can see why many of the sleep problems we face are driven by a world that is always on, and days that lack intentional moments of restoration and relaxation.

That said, not all sleep disruption is simply a lifestyle issue. There are several common sleep disorders that show up in clinical practice, and recognising their patterns matter, because persistent sleep problems often require more than just 'better habits'.

The three most prevalent sleep disorders are:

- insomnia
- obstructive sleep apnoea
- restless legs syndrome.

Each disrupts sleep in a different way, but all can significantly impact energy, focus, mood and daytime functioning if left unaddressed.

Insomnia

Insomnia is the most common sleep disorder and is defined as ongoing difficulty falling asleep, staying asleep or waking too early with daytime impairment.

Insomnia is often about a nervous system that is stuck in 'on' mode and struggles to power down. Stress, workload, life transitions, pain, illness and inconsistent routines all drive hyperarousal, and worry about not sleeping keeps the brain even more alert.

The best-supported treatment is cognitive behavioural therapy for insomnia (CBT-I), which major guidelines recommend as first-line care, and which outperforms sleep medication over the long term when combined with consistent sleep-wake routines.[87]

When worry keeps you awake with guest expert Dr Maria-Elena Lukeides

Dr. Maria-Elena Lukeides is a doctorate-trained clinical psychologist with over 25 years of experience helping people move through emotional pain and unlock their deeper potential. She works across a wide range of concerns, including depression, anxiety, OCD, insomnia, trauma and panic. Her approach blends evidence-based psychological therapies with insights from neuroscience, behavioural design, evolutionary psychology, and somatic practices.

Most of us have had a few restless nights, but insomnia is something quite different. It's when trouble falling asleep, staying asleep or waking too early happens several nights each week and starts to affect daily life. Chronic insomnia lasts for months and often doesn't respond to typical sleep hygiene techniques alone.

In my experience working with people over the years, chronic insomnia is often less about sleep itself and more about the anxiety that surrounds it. After a few bad nights, the thought of another sleepless one can feel unbearable. The frustration of being tired but unable to rest creates stress and activates our adrenaline system—and you can't sleep while your body believes it needs to stay alert. Sleep and self-protection simply don't coexist.

Here's the paradox: sleep only comes when we stop trying to make it happen. Sleep is not something we do, it's something that happens when we let go. You don't consciously digest food or make your heart beat—it happens automatically, and so does sleep. Our job is to create the right environment and ease off the effort. When we're in a state of 'non-doing', sleep returns on its own. Think of unwinding as creating space for sleep to arrive. Watching something light and familiar (a gentle sitcom or favourite old series) helps soothe the mind because it doesn't demand effort or concentration. I often joke that *Brooklyn Nine-Nine* is my favourite sleeping pill; my daughter and I rarely make it past the first few minutes before drifting off.

In contrast, scrolling on your phone or watching something new keeps your brain switched on and alert, which is the opposite of what's needed. Effort, attention and excitement all signal 'wake up', not 'rest'. Over time, many people begin to associate bedtime with wakefulness. The mind treats it as prime time for thinking, planning or replaying the day's worries. Even if you fall asleep, you might wake to a flood of intrusive thoughts. Catastrophic beliefs about sleep, like 'I won't cope tomorrow if I don't sleep', can make matters worse, leading to caffeine overuse, daytime fatigue and even more anxiety. When insomnia becomes persistent, combining acceptance with evidence-based strategies such as the following is most effective.

Stimulus control therapy

Reserve your bed for sleep and intimacy only. Go to bed when you're genuinely sleepy. If you're still awake after about 20 minutes, get up and do something quiet and relaxing until the next wave of sleepiness arrives. Avoid checking the time—it only creates pressure. No matter how little you sleep, wake up at the same time each morning. This consistency helps reset your body clock.

Sleep restriction therapy

Temporarily limit time in bed to roughly the number of hours you're actually sleeping, then gradually extend it as your sleep becomes deeper and more consistent. This may feel tough at first, but it helps rebuild a strong sleep drive and reduces time spent awake in bed.

Cognitive therapy for insomnia

Notice unhelpful thoughts like 'I can't function if I don't sleep' and replace them with gentler alternatives: 'Tomorrow may be hard, but I'll manage once the day gets going.' Remember, our bodies are remarkably resilient and will sleep when they truly need to. Trust in that built-in wisdom.

Mindfulness and relaxation training

Mindful breathing, progressive muscle relaxation or body-scan meditations help calm the nervous system and ease the mind away from repetitive thoughts. These practices don't cause sleep, they invite it. Acceptance and calm pave the way for rest.

Finally, if sleeplessness persists, it's important to check in with a healthcare professional. Insomnia often accompanies conditions such as depression, anxiety, chronic pain, restless leg syndrome or sleep apnoea. But the good news is that, with a mix of acceptance, gentle discipline and trust in your body's natural rhythm, sleep has a way of finding its way back—quietly, naturally, and often when you stop trying so hard.

Obstructive sleep apnoea

Obstructive sleep apnoea occurs when the airway narrows or collapses during sleep, causing breathing to stop and start repeatedly throughout the night. This often comes with loud snoring, gasping or choking sounds, although many people are unaware it is happening.

Each time breathing pauses, the body briefly wakes just enough to reopen the airway. These micro-arousals can happen dozens or even hundreds of times a night, resulting in sleep that never feels restorative.

Left untreated, sleep apnoea increases the risk of high blood pressure, cardiovascular disease, metabolic issues and significant daytime sleepiness. Diagnosis usually involves a sleep study, and treatment may include CPAP therapy, lifestyle changes or other medical interventions, depending on the individual.[88]

Restless legs syndrome

Restless legs syndrome is characterised by uncomfortable sensations in the legs and a strong urge to move them, particularly in the evening or at night when resting. It is often described as crawling, tingling, pulling or 'restless' feelings that make it hard to lie still.

Symptoms typically worsen at rest and improve temporarily with movement, which can delay sleep onset and lead to repeated disruption through the night. Restless legs syndrome can be linked to iron deficiency, pregnancy, certain medications or genetic factors.

Treatment depends on the underlying cause and may include correcting iron levels or using medications that reduce nerve-related symptoms.[89]

Sleep better to eat better

I've already touched on how what you eat impacts your sleep, but what is often overlooked is how quickly sleep feeds back into what you are driven to eat.

Even one or two nights of inadequate sleep can shift appetite regulation. Hunger signals increase, fullness cues weaken and your desire for quick, energy-dense foods becomes stronger.

After just one night of poor sleep, your brain becomes more reactive to high-calorie foods, while the regions responsible for self-control are dialled down. Even without feeling hungrier, you can be drawn more strongly to energy-dense foods and can consume up to 600 extra calories the following day.[90]

This is exactly why established rhythms matter. When you are operating from a set of consistent behaviours rather than how you feel, which changes in a sleep-deprived state, you reduce reliance on willpower and reactive choices.

A word on sleep supplements

Supplements are not a replacement for the sleep fundamentals and routines that make up your sleep rhythm, but they can play a supportive role once your sleep rhythm has been improved. Before commencing, if you have any medical conditions, take regular medications or have concerns about interactions, please seek advice from your GP or another qualified health professional before starting any sleep-related supplement.

Magnesium

Magnesium is involved in nervous system regulation, and research suggests small improvements in insomnia symptoms and sleep onset latency with oral magnesium, particularly in people with low baseline sleep quality. A recent study found that 1 g per day of magnesium L-threonate for 21 days improved objective deep and REM sleep scores and subjective sleep quality and daytime functioning compared to placebo in adults with self-reported sleep problems.[91] Early data on magnesium bisglycinate also shows modest reductions in insomnia severity in adults with poor sleep.[92]

Tart cherry

Tart cherry contains naturally occurring melatonin and polyphenols, and small clinical studies suggest that regular consumption of tart cherry juice can modestly increase sleep duration and improve sleep quality, particularly in people with disrupted sleep.[93] In healthy adults and in those with insomnia, short-term supplementation has been shown to increase total sleep and sleep efficiency and may slightly shorten the time it takes to fall asleep.[94] Fun fact: tart cherry is also commonly used in sports settings, as some research has shown it can modestly reduce post-exercise muscle soreness and markers of exercise-induced muscle damage.[95]

Apigenin

Apigenin is a plant compound found naturally in foods like chamomile and parsley, and is being studied for its potential calming effects. Early human work with apigenin-rich chamomile extracts in people with chronic insomnia shows modest improvements in some sleep measures, including daytime functioning.[96]

Creatine

The research in this space is exciting, with promising evidence that creatine may help mitigate the cognitive effects of sleep deprivation using both a long-term, low daily dose and a single high-dose strategy. A one-off high dose of creatine (0.35 grams per kilogram of body weight) taken during prolonged sleep deprivation has been shown to partially offset the usual decline in cognitive performance and processing speed, with brain imaging suggesting a buffering effect on mental fatigue.[97] That same dose comes with a clear warning: this is not something to trial casually, as high doses can cause significant gastrointestinal upset if you are not already tolerating a regular baseline intake.

More practically, daily dosing of around 5 grams appears far more relevant for most people. Longer term supplementation at these doses can increase brain creatine stores and has been associated with better performance on demanding cognitive tasks, particularly when the brain is stressed, for example, under sleep loss or high mental load.[98] For most, this offers a safer, more sustainable way to build brain creatine reserves over time and improve resilience to common short-sleep nights caused by work pressure or travel, without relying on experimental high-dose protocols.

Knowing when to investigate further

It is important to acknowledge that some sleep disruption warrants further investigation. While many everyday sleep issues sit within habits, timing and recovery, there are situations where medical contributors need to be considered. Conditions such as sleep apnoea, restless legs syndrome, hormonal or thyroid imbalances, chronic pain and mental health conditions can all significantly interfere with sleep quality, regardless of how well someone manages their routine.

If sleep remains consistently unrefreshing despite good sleep habits, or if symptoms such as loud snoring, gasping during sleep, frequent night waking, persistent early waking or excessive daytime sleepiness are present, it is worth investigating further. Your GP is the best starting point, and they can assess whether a referral to a sleep physician, psychologist or another relevant specialist is appropriate.

Activity

Reflect on these questions to complete your sleep rhythm audit:

- What time do I wake up and go to bed on weekdays and weekends?
- What time do I have my last coffee or caffeine-based drink? Is it more or less than eight to nine hours before bed?
- What time do I have dinner? How close to your bedtime is it?
- When do I switch off from screens (TV, laptops, phones etc)?
- Would a go-to-bed alarm (page 176) help protect my sleep window?
- What do I currently do before I go to bed? Do I have a set routine I follow each night (weekdays and weekends)?

Now, choose one behaviour from your answers that feels easiest to improve and commit to that to start work on your sleep rhythm.

Conclusion

Sleep is the foundation for how you show up today, tomorrow and in the future. When your sleep is restorative, your capacity to do more and take on more is automatically expanded. If sleep is something you struggle with, or you have accepted you just 'don't sleep that well', it's time to rewrite that narrative.

Getting a good night's sleep starts long before your head hits the pillow. It starts with regulating the time you wake in the morning, early daylight exposure, being consistent with your nutrition rhythm, eliminating external cues, and allowing for moments of relaxation and reflection across the day so your brain has space to process it before you jump into bed.

When you start to elevate or embed behaviours that improve your sleep rhythm, commit to them consistently and protect these standards at all costs, sleep becomes the foundation for one of the most powerful levers to elevating your energy, recovery, wellbeing and performance.

Chapter Eight

Connection—With your values, your purpose and your people

Human beings are physically wired for belonging. As a species, we survived by being in groups. Belonging meant protection, shared labour, food and care. In comparison, being isolated usually meant danger. That evolutionary reality still shapes how our biology responds today. Strong social connections act as a safety signal, whereas loneliness and social isolation are treated by the brain and body as a chronic stressor.[99]

Your body and brain are constantly scanning your environment for safety or threat cues, and other people are one of the strongest signals. When you feel socially connected, supported and understood, your physiology reflects this with lower stress hormones, better immune function, lower levels of inflammatory markers and improved sleep quality.

When connection is strained or missing, your system shifts in the opposite direction. Your stress response stays switched on longer; sleep is impacted; inflammatory markers rise; mood, focus and cognitive function decline. Over time, this is associated with higher risk of chronic disease and earlier health decline.

Large-scale research shows that people with stronger social relationships live longer than those who are more socially isolated, with effects similar in size to other major health risk factors.[100] More recently, the WHO Commission on Social Connection (2025) estimated that social disconnection affects around one in six people worldwide, and contributes to reduced life expectancy on a scale similar to smoking or air pollution.[101]

Connection also shapes how we experience stress and pain. Studies show that social rejection activates overlapping regions with physical pain, which helps explain why relationship stress can affect sleep, mood, focus and energy.[102]

For this fifth rhythm, connection refers to both how you relate to others and how connected you feel to yourself—including your values and sense of purpose.

Connection isn't one thing, it has many layers. There is connection to yourself where you feel grounded in your values, your needs and what matters most. There is connection to your inner circle, the people who matter most in your life. There is connection to community, where you feel part of something bigger. And there is connection at work, where you feel supported, seen and not like you have to carry everything.

Having a reason to contribute, belong and matter changes how effort is experienced. When life feels meaningful, challenge is easier to tolerate. When meaning is missing, even small demands can feel heavy. Research shows that people who report higher levels of purpose have better mental health, greater resilience to stress and lower risk of early death. Purpose shapes behaviour, but it also appears to shape stress biology and inflammation directly.[103]

Community strengthens this effect. Strong social bonds buffer stress, support recovery and protect against long-term health decline, with an impact on mortality comparable to many traditional health behaviours. This pattern shows up clearly in the world's 'blue zones', where people live longer and stay healthier for more of their lives. While diet and movement matter, one of the strongest common threads is community. Belonging is daily life through family, friendships, shared rituals and regular social contact.[104]

Purpose and community are part of the structure that allows humans to carry load over time. When both are strong, pressure is easier to bear. When they are weak, the same pressure becomes harder to sustain.

In this chapter, you will see why connection is the fifth rhythm in your daily operating system.

Social connection buffers stress

Two people can carry the same workload, face the same deadlines and live with the same responsibilities. One feels stretched but stable; the other feels constantly on edge. The difference is not discipline or toughness, it is capacity.

Social connection is a powerful lever for expanding capacity by buffering stress. When social support is present, the physiological stress response is dampened, allowing the body to recover more efficiently and reducing the cumulative load stress places on us.[105]

Your nervous system is like a 24-hour security system, constantly scanning for safety or threat cues. Other people are one of the strongest signals it looks for. We learn this early. In childhood, caregivers act as powerful stress regulators, shaping how the nervous system learns to settle in the presence of support. Over time, that role shifts to friends, partners and trusted others.

When connection is present, our stress response resolves more easily. We're able to better return to a baseline. When connection is missing or strained, stress remains activated for longer, recovery takes more time and the same demands feel heavier than they otherwise would.[106]

This is why managing stress is not only about building in recovery pulses, and controlling your workload, schedules and habits. Who you are connected to, and how deeply, shapes your stress tolerance over time.

Values and purpose

Effort feels different when it is attached to something that matters. You can work long hours, carry big responsibility and tolerate pressure when you believe in what you are doing. But when your days are filled with tasks that feel disconnected from your values, the same workload feels heavier due to a lack of meaning.[107]

Simon Sinek captured this in *Start With Why* when he wrote, 'People don't buy what you do, they buy why you do it'. The same is true of your own nervous system. It does not just respond to what you are doing, it responds to why you are doing it.

Purpose acts like a filter. It changes how stress is interpreted. When what you are doing aligns with what you care about, challenge feels purposeful. When it does not, the same challenge feels pointless, draining and harder to recover from. Reframing challenge through a sense of meaning or purpose can reduce how stressful demands feel and is one way you can buffer the impact of stress on your health.[108]

This is why two people can live very similar lives and feel very differently about them. One feels tired but fulfilled; the other feels tired and empty. Values give context to effort. They answer: *Why is this worth it?*

When that answer is clear, pressure becomes something you can engage with. When it is unclear, pressure becomes something you simply endure.

You see this most clearly when people reach goals they thought would fix everything. It might look like a promotion, the business growing, the recognition coming—and, instead of feeling grounded, they feel flat. Success without alignment does not fulfil us, so instead, the goal posts move and we turn out attention to 'the next thing'.

Sinek also wrote, 'Working hard for something we do not care about is called stress. Working hard for something we love is called passion.' That statement describes how meaning changes the way effort is processed.

Misalignment creates a different kind of fatigue. You can eat well, train well and sleep well and still feel flat if what you are doing all day quietly contradicts what you care about. This is something I learnt the hard way. When I was giving everything I had (and then some) to my job, I was operating out of misalignment. At first it felt amazing, but over time, as I added more teams and gave more of myself to everyone else than I did my own life, the cost started to show. Over the years, it wore me down, both from the unsustainable workload and mental load that I had taken on. Health is my number one value, and a big part of that is managing stress and recovery, which I was neglecting.

Reflection

Here are some questions you might like to reflect or journal on:

- Where are you saying 'yes' to things that cost more than they give?
- Where are you performing well but feeling empty?
- Where does your life look good on paper but feel wrong in your body?

Purpose is a form of connection: connection to what you care about, connection to something bigger than your to-do list, connection to a reason that makes the load worth carrying. If you are not sure where to start when it comes to identifying your values and living in alignment with them, you are not alone. I felt the same for a long time. That is why I worked with someone to learn how to do this properly.

Read through the following list of values and pay attention to what stands out. Start by choosing ten values that speak to you, then narrow them down to your top five. This is by no means an exhaustive list of values, but it is enough to get you started if this is something new to you.

Achievement
Adaptability
Adventure
Ambition
Balance
Commitment
Consistency
Courage
Curiosity
Discipline
Energy
Excellence
Family
Friendship
Fun
Growth
Happiness
Health
Integrity
Leadership
Longevity
Ownership
Peace
Personal development
Pleasure
Relationships
Resilience
Responsibility
Simplicity
Sustainability
Wealth
Wellbeing

Once you've picked your five values, reflect on how they show up in your life right now. Where are you living in alignment with them, and where are you not? And, if you truly lived by these values, how might the way you make decisions, the way you structure your days, and the way you set your priorities begin to change?

This is not a set-and-forget exercise. Your values can (and should) be revisited regularly. I review mine yearly with my end-of-year reflection. Some will stay the same, and some will evolve as you do.

In my 20s and early 30s, I was driven by achievement. Work hard, say 'yes' to everything—ambition, excellence, growth and leadership were all driving me. Health mattered, it always has, but the narrative I carried at the time was 'I can do it all'. If there was more to take on, I took it. If there was a higher bar, I chased it. My sense of worth became closely tied to output, to what I could build, win or achieve.

Those values weren't wrong. They helped me create a career, a reputation and a business I am proud of. But they came with a cost. There was very little room for fun, joy, friends (outside of work) or real relaxation, and over time, that felt like living out of alignment. It all came to a head when I became really unwell for 12 to 18 months. I was exhausted, bedbound for days and weeks on end. After extensive investigations, with multiple specialists, we realised it was years of burnout plus long COVID-19 all rolled into one.

When your health is jeopardised, it really makes one thing clear—with your health you can have a thousand goals, without it, you have one. That period forced me to really confront how I had been operating and what it was really costing me. I remember one moment clearly. The NSW Waratahs wanted me to run their Performance Nutrition Program at the end of 2019. I was sitting in the Giants Netball office talking to one of their staff, and I remember saying to her, 'I genuinely don't know if I can learn another 50 athletes' and staff names'. But I said 'yes' anyway, despite knowing it was too much and I was already beyond capacity.

When COVID-19 hit in March 2020, the world stopped. And, for the first time in a long time, so did I. It gave me space to get honest with myself, not just about my health, but about my life—my relationships, my energy, my ability to enjoy what I had built and achieved.

For the first time, I had to ask not just *can* I do this, but *is it worth it*?

COVID-19 caused chaos in professional sport. Contracts were paused or reduced. It was stressful, but it also forced a realisation I wasn't expecting. I had built my identity around being needed, always being 'on' and my job title. And yet, the moment this happened, I felt disposable.

That combination was a turning point. It made me step back and reassess the last ten to 15 years of how I'd been operating, and what I wanted the next decade or two to look and feel like. In doing that, one thing became clear: I had no boundaries.

People learn what to expect from you based on the conditions you set, and the conditions I set were simple: I am always on, always available, and I will go above and beyond. That was exhausting, and I needed to change that moving forward. I didn't walk away from the sports team contracts overnight, but I did get clear on an exit plan. I also got clear that I was no longer willing to give everything to my work.

That shift required support and identity work, and that's when I reached out to life coach Shannah Kennedy after I interviewed her on my first podcast, *my millennial health*. Working with her helped me see patterns clearly, shift my focus from business to myself, and identify my values and how I could live in alignment with them.

Now, in my late 30s, my values look different again, as does my life. I am now a mother (my little girl just turned one a few weeks ago), I've left a business that was no longer aligned with my vision and values, and I've built a new one that reflects who I am now.

In this season, I want more space in my days and weeks, more ease, more flow and more energy. I want more time with my little girl, as I know it will go so fast, and some time for myself to do what matters to me. I still care about excellence, about impact and about doing meaningful work, but I care just as much about how I feel doing it, and how much of my life it takes up.

To be clear, I loved my time in professional sport. I worked with incredible athletes and staff, many of whom I still have amazing relationships with today. I was part of premierships, championships and grand finals. I built relationships that will stay with me for life. It was a dream I'd had since I was a teenager, but I no longer work inside team environments. These days, I primarily speak at events, run programs with leaders, emerging leaders and organisations, host my podcast *Stay at the Top* and work with a limited number of private coaching clients. While, today, I mainly work with executives and leaders, it has also included elite athletes such as Rohan Browning, James Magnussen, Errol Gulden, Josh Kelly, Dane Rampe and Keesja Gofers.

But as life does, I evolved, and my values evolved too. That is what values do, which is why it's important to revisit them. When your values and the decisions you make reflect who you are and what matters, your boundaries become easier to enforce and everything feels more effortless as it is in alignment with what truly matters to you. This is the definition of the path of least resistance. Green flags!

Connection has layers

So, how do you know when your connection rhythm is off?

For many of us, it shows up as subtle disconnection at first. You might notice that you:

- feel flat when your nutrition, exercise, recovery and sleep are pretty good
- are surrounded by people, but still feel lonely or not understood
- stop reaching out, even to people you care about
- are more irritable, less patient and more reactive than usual
- feel like you're carrying everything yourself
- have lost your sense of fun, lightness and perspective
- don't feel like yourself and you can't explain why.

Consider these signals that reflect how your connection rhythm is going.

A word on boundaries

Boundaries are something many of us struggle with, and I get it, I struggled with them for a long time too. But we need to reframe what boundaries actually are. They are not about being difficult or selfish, they are about protecting your energy, so you can show up properly for the things and people who matter most.

Think about the safety demonstration on a plane. You're always told to put your own oxygen mask on first before helping anyone else. Hopefully, you never need to do it, but the principle is important. If you run out of air, you're no help to anyone. The same rule applies in real life. And here's the part most people miss—when you prioritise yourself, it doesn't just benefit you, it benefits everyone around you: your family, your team, your clients, your colleagues.

This is one of the biggest struggles I see people face. And don't get me wrong, it comes from a place of good intentions. But when you put your family, your team, your business, your career ahead of yourself, you unintentionally put yourself last. No one is immune to it. I've seen it across all ages, roles and industries. I have run workshops, delivered keynotes and coached some of the country's most well-known CEOs, and even some of them struggle!

What helps is a simple reframe: when I say 'yes' to this, what am I saying 'no' to?

Often the 'no' is to one of the following: time, energy, sleep, presence, health or yourself.

And, most of the time, it isn't intentional. Most of us are not choosing to put ourselves last. But when we keep saying 'yes' to everyone else, without our own operating system in place that we're proactive and intentional with, we end up unintentionally saying 'no' to ourselves.

I was a 'yes' person for most of my life. Professionally, as I have spoken about before, but personally too. I loved being busy, being needed, being on the go. Saying 'yes' felt like opportunity, connection, success.

But part of that was also avoidance. If I stayed busy enough, I did not have to listen to what I was tired of, what I needed or what was no longer working. Boundaries forced me to get honest and clear on what I needed.

They showed me that every 'yes' is a trade, and not every trade is worth it.

If your life does not reflect what you say you care about (your values), part of the reason might be your boundaries (or lack thereof). Like anything, the more we do something the easier it gets. I think a lot less about a 'no, thank you' now than I did before. I don't have to over explain it, like I used to, and the same will happen for you if this is something you struggle with.

Relationship quality and long-term health

Which of the following do you think has the biggest impact on your long-term wellbeing?

- What you eat
- How you move your body
- How you manage your stress and recover
- How you sleep
- The quality of your relationships.

While all are important, one of the longest running studies, the Harvard Study of Adult Development, which has followed people for more than 80 years, has shown that the quality of your relationships is the biggest predictor of your health and longevity.

The Harvard study has found that those who report warm, trusting relationships live longer, stay mentally sharper and experience less chronic disease. People who feel lonely or disconnected are more likely to become unwell earlier, even when their lifestyle looks good on paper. This research showed that relationship quality at 50 predicted health at 80 better than cholesterol, IQ or genes.[109]

Psychiatrist Robert Waldinger, who currently leads the study, shared these findings in his TED Talk *What Makes a Good Life? Lessons from the longest study on happiness*, which has now been viewed by tens of millions of people around the world (nearly 29 million at time of writing!).[110]

The message from more than eight decades of data is clear: *Good relationships keep us happier and healthier.*

Waldinger summarises three big lessons.

1. Social connection is good for us. Loneliness is not just sad, it is harmful. People who are more connected to family, friends and community live longer.
2. It is not the number of relationships that matters, but the quality. Living in the middle of constant conflict or emotional distance is damaging to health, even if you are not technically alone.
3. Good relationships protect both the body and the brain. People who feel securely supported by their partner in later life stay mentally sharper for longer.

He also clarified that relationships are not always neat or easy. They are messy, emotional and sometimes inconvenient. They can be lifelong, and they matter more than anything else we chase, add or focus on. Your friends, family and community are fundamental to the quality of your health and life.

So, what does this mean for you? It means going deeper where it counts and where it feels right for you, which differs from person to person, depending on where you sit on the extrovert and introvert scale. But some ideas might include:

- replacing some screen time with real connection
- creating a recurring ritual like a weekly walk, a coffee catch up or a Sunday meal

- doing something new together: walks, shared meals, simple routines, date nights
- reaching out to someone you have lost touch with or have fallen out with.

This really takes the idea of you being the sum of the five people you spend the most time with to a whole new level!

Lessons from the longest-living populations

When people talk about living longer, the focus usually goes to food, exercise, sleep or genetics. And, yes, all of those things matter. But when researchers look at the places in the world where people live the longest and stay the healthiest for more of their lives, one pattern keeps showing up: *community*. Enter the Blue Zones.

Blue Zones

When Dan Buettner set out to find the world's longest-living people, he identified regions where people were far more likely to live into their 90s and 100s, and then went to see how they actually lived. What he found became known as Blue Zones.

While on the surface, the people in these Blue Zones are from different cultures, eat different foods and keep to different routines, clear patterns began to emerge, and one of the strongest threads running through every long-living region was *connection*.

In many long-living cultures (such as Okinawa, Japan; Sardinia, Italy; Ikaria, Greece; and Nicoya, Costa Rica), people do not age alone. Older adults remain embedded in family and community life, with connection and contribution woven into everyday routines.

This matters because sustained connection gives people an ongoing role and a reason to stay engaged. Purpose does not disappear with age or retirement. They contribute by caring for grandchildren, tending gardens, preparing food and participating in daily life. This sense of 'I still matter' shapes how people experience ageing.

Meals are rarely rushed and rarely eaten alone. People eat together. They talk, laugh and argue. Ultimately, what this means at a biological level is: *I belong*. That sense of belonging shapes who you believe you are.

How identity forms

You do not build your sense of self in isolation. Who you are is shaped in relationships. From early life, identity is formed through being seen, reflected and responded to. We learn who we are through how others meet us. Over time, that becomes an internal story: this is who I am, this is where I fit, this is how I matter.

Belonging stabilises that story. When you know where you belong, you do not have to keep proving who you are.[111]

When belonging is thin or conditional, our identity becomes fragile. We start using performance as proof. That can look like achievement, productivity, being useful, being impressive. For a while that works, until the role changes, the title shifts, the season or career ends. Performance-based self-worth like this is consistently associated with more stress and higher risk of burnout.[112] This is why some people can feel lost after success, retirement, injury, redundancy or burnout.

The modern disconnection problem

How many ways do you communicate with your friends? Let me guess. There is Instagram or TikTok for memes and reels, a WhatsApp group chat, the iMessage thread, Facebook for events and invites. Does that sound about right? I know it is for me.

On paper, we have never been more connected. We can message anyone at any time, work from almost anywhere, and stay in touch across countries and time zones. And yet, loneliness and social disconnection are rising. Something in the way we now live is not matching what we actually need as human beings, and there are a few factors at play.

Remote and hybrid work

Remote and hybrid work have changed how many of us live and work. For some of us, it has created freedom and flexibility; for others, it has quietly removed the small moments of human contact that once came built into the day: the hallway chats, shared coffee breaks, quick vents. When those disappear, work can become efficient but emotionally thin. You still get things done, but you do it alone or it takes a Zoom call for a quick check-in or collaboration.[113]

Research in remote workers shows that greater loneliness and poorer emotional regulation are strongly linked to higher depression, anxiety and stress, with more days working remotely increasing anxiety partly through a reduced ability to regulate emotions.[114]

The solution is not necessarily a return to the office part-time or full time, and for some people that is not an option. But, if connection is no longer built into your workday, it's about being aware of this, and looking at how you can design it somewhere else.

If you work remote or hybrid, ask yourself:

- Where is my regular face-to-face contact coming from?
- Who do I see consistently each week?
- Where do I feel part of something, not just working on my own?
- Where do I have conversations that go beyond task and transaction?

That might be a co-working space once or twice a week, a training group, a cafe, a standing breakfast with a friend or colleague, or even relocating certain meetings to in-person catch ups.

For me, with the type of work I now do, and with my young daughter, unless I am meeting someone face-to-face or presenting at an event, I am home a lot more. I realised I was missing a lot of incidental connection, so I joined a space where I can work from that also has events and a wellness facility. It gives structure to my week, and a place to work, enjoy and connect outside of the home.

Social media

Social media adds another layer. It offers the appearance of connection without the biology of it. You see people, react, scroll and comment, but your nervous system does not register that in the same way it reads and responds to real presence. There is no shared physical space, no tone of voice, no full range of non-verbal cues. Many of the signals that normally help calm us are muted or missing.[115]

On top of that, social media often adds comparison. You see the highlights reel, which is often what others are doing, achieving or becoming without their doubts, fatigue or mess. The book *Comparisonitis*, by Melissa Ambrosini, captures this well, showing how social media amplifies our urge to keep up with others and constantly measure our lives against what we see in our feeds.

The answer isn't to delete your accounts or go on a social media detox—I mean you can, but the reality is this is the world we now live in, and as you know, I am not about extremes as they rarely last.

The real shift is awareness. Social media can supplement connection, but it does not replace it. Treat social media as an addition not a substitute. Prioritise real conversations, shared experiences and time with people in real life, or if they live far away, pick up the phone!

Social media is an area I always want to reduce my time on, because when does it ever make you feel better about yourself? For me, I have rules around when I use it. I do not consume in the morning, and I do not scroll close to bedtime. Having a stand in the kitchen where my phone sleeps helps me stick to that.

Activity

If you haven't already, go through the Values activity on page 196 and identify ten values. Then sit with these and reduce them to your top five. Pull out a journal or notes app on your phone and write these values in order of priority and why they are important to you.

Reflect on how you have been living, and whether you have been in alignment with these values. Identify where you have and where you haven't.

Then use one of my favourite frameworks to think about what you are going to start, stop and keep doing to live more in alignment with your values:

- I am going to start doing ...
- I am going to stop doing ...
- I am going to keep doing ...

Conclusion

Connection is not nice to have, it's a biological requirement. Your nervous system is constantly scanning for safety or threat, and the quality of your relationships is one of the strongest signals it receives.

When you feel supported, understood and like you belong, your body downregulates stress more efficiently. When connection is missing or strained, your stress response stays switched on for longer, recovery is slower and the same demands or challenges feel harder than they otherwise would.

This rhythm is multi-layered. It includes how connected you feel to yourself through your values, purpose and identity, and how connected you are to the people around you. Your other four rhythms can be established, but if this rhythm isn't, your body and brain can feel and show this missing piece.

The goal is to still be intentional and live in alignment with who you are. Build and invest in relationships that are warm, trusting and real and protect your boundaries. Sustainable high performance is built through a sense of belonging.

Social connection and the quality of relationships are fundamental to our physical and mental health.

Chapter Nine

Getting your operating system up and running

My intention with this book has always been simple. As you read through it, I want you to reflect on what you are already doing well; get clear on where your opportunities for improvement sit across your five rhythms; and have a reliable, easy-to-digest companion that gives you a clear roadmap for building your own daily operating system.

Most importantly, this book is not about copying someone else's routine or operating system. It is about giving you the tools to select the habits that best fit your rhythms, demands and season of life, so your operating system is truly tailored to you.

I also know what tends to happen at this point in a book like this: you feel motivated and energised to change everything all at once. Despite the reminder to focus on one behaviour and one rhythm at a time, it can feel tempting to overhaul ten things immediately. I get it.

This is exactly why this chapter exists. Before we move into how your operating system flexes when you travel for work or life, move through busy seasons, or hit periods where the usual habits no longer fit, this is your moment to pause, and get clear on your path forward.

At its core, your daily operating system for sustainable performance serves three key functions that we covered in Chapter 1:

1. Charge up: How you create and sustain energy
2. Capacity: How you build your stress tolerance and resilience
3. Charge down: How you wind down and effectively recover.

These functions are created by the five key rhythms that make up your daily operating system:

1. Nutrition
2. Exercise
3. Stress and recovery
4. Sleep
5. Connection.

Each rhythm is made up of one or more behaviours. And it is these behaviours, chosen deliberately and practised proactively and consistently, that shape how you feel, perform and recover each day.

Depending on where you are starting from, this might feel like a significant rebuild, or it might be just a few strategic upgrades. Either way, my recommendation is the same: start slow and start small.

Decades of behaviour change research shows that tiny, specific actions repeated consistently are far more likely to become automatic habits than big overhauls.[116] Choose one behaviour from one rhythm, focus on that, and stick with it until it feels like second nature, then move on to the next behaviour or rhythm.

Stabilising your daily operating system

Up until now, this book has helped you understand the rhythms and behaviours that make up your daily operating system. This is where we turn that understanding into action.

The goal here is to choose a clear starting point and build from there. Across each of the five rhythms, ask yourself one question: *What is the one habit that would make the biggest difference for me right now and that feels like the path of least resistance?*

Once you have clarity on the key behaviour for each rhythm, think about which function of your daily operating system it serves.

- Will this behaviour help you create or sustain more energy?
- Will it help expand your capacity and build your stress tolerance?
- Will it help you downshift and recover more effectively?

Some behaviours may serve more than one function, which is a bonus.

At this point, you will likely have a long list of ideas, upgrades and habits you want to embed. That is totally fine and normal, but this is where focus matters. Behaviour change research shows that trying to change too many behaviours at once makes it harder for any single change to become automatic, whereas narrowing your attention to a small number of specific actions and repeating them supports habit formation.[117]

The priority now is to distil your list of five behaviours across the five rhythms to a few behaviours to begin with. Three is the maximum, but one is often enough.

As a guide, research on habit formation suggests that, for many health behaviours, automaticity typically builds over a period of roughly two to five months, with simpler actions developing more quickly and more complex routines taking longer, and with considerable individual variability.

So, with that in mind, please give yourself at least two to four weeks of consistent practice with your chosen behaviour (or behaviours) before you layer on the next upgrade or focus on another rhythm.[118]

By starting with one or two core behaviours, you will feel a huge difference to your energy, recovery and overall performance. Tune in to the subjective metric that matters most to you (that you identified in Chapter 2), and use that as your daily reference point on how things are tracking.

Anchors that hold the system together

When life changes, your operating system needs something to hold onto. Anchors are the behaviours that keep your system intact, regardless of what else is going on in your life.

Anchors are the behaviours you return to when your week is full, plans change or your day doesn't go as you thought it would. Without anchors, it is easy to feel like you are off track, or you've 'fallen off the wagon'. You haven't—life happens.

Anchors allow your operating system to adapt and go with the chaos of life, without losing your entire system.

Your domino habit

The most important anchor in your operating system is your domino habit. This is the first behaviour you do that sets the tone for the rest of your day. For some people, it is exercising or meditating first thing in the morning; for others it's a high-protein breakfast, or hydrating with water or electrolytes before their morning coffee. I once had someone tell me after a panel event that their domino habit was meeting a friend before work for a coffee. It's completely unique to you.

The point is, when it happens, your day runs more smoothly. Decisions feel easier, your energy is more stable, you move from task to task easier. Green flags!

This is your domino habit.

When you miss this habit, everything takes more effort, you feel like you are playing catch up all day, and you expend more cognitive energy and bandwidth to make things happen.

For most of us, our domino habit sits first thing in the morning. Early in the day, you have more control, fewer competing demands and schedule changes, and more space to act intentionally.

Ideally, your domino habit is something you can do on any day and in any situation, regardless of whether it is a workday in the office, at home, on the road, in an airport lounge etc.

Take some time to reflect on what your domino habit is and whether it is the same for different contexts.

Reflection

- What is your domino habit at home?
- What is your domino habit when you are in the office?
- What is it when you are travelling?

Your domino habit helps you move from living reactively to being proactive. All you need to do is identify it and protect it. Just like the first domino in a row, once it falls, the rest of the day tends to follow more effortlessly. Here's an example.

Case study: Identifying your domino habit

Rob is an entrepreneur and leads a team of hundreds of staff. His work is social by nature — part of that is the job, part of it is just who he has always been. But now, in his late 30s, he is at a crossroads.

He doesn't want to be known as 'fun Rob' anymore. He wants to be 'fit Rob', because he knows that shift will ripple into every part of his life. It will change how he shows up as a founder, a leader and a father.

When we first started working together, he was all in. He trained most days, ate a high-protein breakfast, made balanced meal choices and prioritised sleep. But as life got busy, everything slowly got more challenging.

So, we stripped it back. We worked out that exercise was his first domino.

When he trained in the morning, everything else followed more effortlessly. Breakfast happened without a second thought. His meals across the day stayed more consistent and dialled in. Sleep got prioritised because his body actually needed it.

Without morning training, everything felt like a conscious decision and a battle. So, his focus shifted to some form of morning movement, and everything else happened more effortlessly, even in his really busy periods.

Another example is a senior executive who now travels less for work and more for pleasure. After working together, she started having electrolytes first thing in the morning before her morning coffee. It became a simple ritual she shared with her husband.

She later went overseas for seven weeks and ordered enough Hyro to take away with her so she could keep that ritual going. That one small habit anchored her mornings, even when everything else around her changed.

Different people, different lives, different domino habits, but the same principle. One behaviour sets the tone for everything that follows. That's your domino habit, and you need to find it and protect it.

Non-negotiables

Alongside your domino habit sits your non-negotiables. These are the absolute minimum combination of habits you commit to on your busiest days. At a minimum, I recommend identifying one non-negotiable that helps you:

- charge up and sustain energy
- charge down and protect your sleep.

You can have more but this is your baseline.

These anchors give your operating system structure regardless of what your day, week or season has in store for you. Clarity on your anchors reduces decision fatigue, protects your energy and helps you stay consistent.

Anchors are what allow your operating system to flex without breaking. They help you live the principle of structured flexibility.

Once these are clear, adapting your system to different seasons, environments and demands becomes far easier, which is what we are moving to next.

Adapting your operating system

Your daily operating system needs to work when life is predictable, and it needs to work when it is not. Up until now, much of this book has focused on what a typical day and week look like, where there is some structure, some routine and enough consistency to build momentum. This all matters as it's your baseline that you will build or adapt from.

But the reality is, life shifts. Maybe you travel for work often, your kids get sick, grandparents are away, work ramps up, deadlines come in thick and fast, plans move, something unexpected happens. The list goes on!

This is where your operating system is tested. The goal in these moments is not to force your usual rhythm to fit if it won't, but to adjust it so it still supports your energy, performance and recovery in a way that works for you right now.

A big part of that is focusing on controlling the controllables.

Control the controllables

This is really about asking yourself one simple question: *What is within my control?*

Elite athletes love this saying! It's ultimately about bringing your focus back to the process and what is within your control—which for an athlete might mean the training they have done, the pre-game meal they had, the extra recovery they did, the visualisation practice they've committed to. What isn't within their control, for example, is the weather or what their opponents have done.

For you, this means that when life happens and chaos follows, you need to bring your attention back to the behaviours you can control in that moment. That shift alone reduces noise, limits unhelpful thinking, conserves energy and helps you stay proactive instead of reactive.

To do this, all you need to do is ask yourself in the moment: *What is within my control right now?* It might be:

- what you eat at breakfast, even if the rest of the day is uncertain
- whether you drink water before coffee
- whether you move your body for ten minutes, even if your normal session is not possible
- whether you get outside and see daylight early.

Start as early in the day as possible

This is one of my universal principles, and it matters even more when your context changes and your usual behaviours and rhythms are disrupted. Whatever you are trying to protect, start it as early in your day as possible.

This is not about being a morning person or forcing an early start. People have different chronotypes and natural rhythms. What matters is anchoring behaviours at the beginning of your day, whenever that is for you.

Early in your day, you typically have more control as all of your competing demands haven't started yet. You also have more cognitive space to act intentionally. As your day unfolds, plans change, fatigue builds and your mind has to deal with more competing interests.

What you do at the start of your day shapes what follows. When movement, food or some structures are anchored early, energy tends to be more stable, appetite is more controlled and decisions later in the day become easier. When that anchor is missed, the cost can show up as low energy, stronger cravings or more reactive choices.

So regardless of where you are, anchor what matters early when it is within your control. If you keep the start of your day as consistent as possible, you are starting from the same foundation each time. This gives your operating system the best chance of holding and running more effortlessly when the rest of the day becomes unpredictable.

This is especially the case if you are travelling for work or life and evenings are social, late and hard to control. Protecting the start of your day helps you stabilise your energy, appetite and decision-making.

Gareth's experience is a good example of how this works in practice.

Case study: Adapting your rhythms

Gareth, a CEO of an accounting company, would travel internationally for work a few times a year. This has historically been a challenge. He would find it hard to maintain a rhythm while he was away, and when he came back, it would take him weeks to get 'back on track'. Part of this was because he didn't have an operating system that adapted while he was away; part of it was his very black-and-white thinking that meant he had unrealistically high expectations of himself while he was away, which was setting him up mentally for failure.

Over the time we worked together, he got clear on what his daily operating system looked like when he was at home, and also how this adapted when he travelled. A big part of it was focusing on the controllables.

For Gareth, even when he travelled, his mornings were predictable, so that became the focus. This was his window to exercise, and he'd prioritise the same high-protein breakfast he had at home regardless of whether he was in a hotel or Airbnb. That was his domino habit. Lunch was generally within his control with a bit of proactive forward planning, which we'd do in his strategy sessions. His afternoons could be unpredictable, but he knew if he went from lunch to dinner, he would turn up to dinner ravenous and he'd be more likely to end up overeating, so he'd aim to have a mid-afternoon snack to help reduce this risk.

Dinner was tricky. It might be with clients or colleagues, and it was generally unpredictable. However, there is a big difference between turning up to dinner ravenous and dehydrated as you've been reactive and completely out of rhythm all day, compared to satisfied, ready to eat but overall in a similar rhythm to normal. If he was in rhythm, or a version of it, he wouldn't overeat as he wasn't starving thanks to his mid-afternoon snack. The flow-on effect of this was huge. He'd finish the night feeling better, have a better sleep and then restart his operating system with his nutrition and exercise rhythm the next day, helping him feel more energised and recovered. Green flags!

This also made returning home and integrating back into his usual operating system easier. Part of that was adjusting his expectations, and staggering his return to his usual operating system. He didn't expect it to just fire back up, day one, with all the jet lag. For him, the initial focus was tactical, like putting meal orders in the week he got back so it was outsourced and he didn't have to think about it. The next was getting some movement in. It didn't have to be straight back to his usual exercise rhythm, instead he embraced progress over perfection.

Tools to support decision-making

Your operating system gives you structure, but there will always be moments when life is busy, plans change or your mental bandwidth is maxed out. Meetings run over, travel disrupts your routine, your diary is stacked with social commitments, and all of a sudden everything feels harder!

Over the years, I have developed some tools I use regularly with clients to support decision-making in these moments. They are not everyday habits or part of your daily operating system, they are practical supports for times when your usual rhythms are disrupted, or you aren't sure what behaviour is best for you.

These tools will help your system bend and flex, rather than break or stop, and make it easier to adapt your behaviours and rhythms.

Run experiments

You might already be familiar with A/B testing, even if you have never called it that. It's what we all do when we try two options and see what works better. Different ways of structuring your day. Different routines that feel easier to stick to.

In business, this approach is common. We test, tweak, measure and refine things like landing pages, marketing campaigns and calls to action in newsletters. When it comes to health, most of us do the opposite. We try something because someone else swears by it and keep going with it without truly assessing if it is working for us.

With your health, if you are not testing, noticing and comparing, you are guessing.

Running experiments simply means changing one thing at a time and paying attention to what happens to important metrics like your energy across the entire day, your stress levels, your appetite, your cravings, your recovery.

If you are going to use this tool, keep your experiments simple and small. Try one version of a habit and then another. Give it two weeks where you change one variable only and check in with how this change is truly impacting you. The case study I shared about Jeff back on page 39 is an example of this. Over time, this builds self-awareness and helps you shape an operating system that actually fits your life, with behaviours that truly work for you.

Tetris

Do you remember Tetris? That game where the blocks fall from the top of the screen and you must rotate and shift them, so they fit together? Sometimes it flows slowly and easily, other times, everything comes at once and you are just trying to keep up.

That is how some days can feel. Tetris is a tool I like to use as an example as it's about adjusting the timing and order of certain behaviours in your day without abandoning your rhythm. You keep the same building blocks, you just move them to fit the day you have ahead of you.

A common example is a meeting close to lunch that you know typically runs over. When this happens, lunch gets pushed back much later than usual or skipped altogether because you go straight into the next meeting.

What I suggest in the future is that you move your afternoon snack to before that next meeting. This way you are keeping a similar nutrition rhythm to what you normally have, with similar time gaps between your meals and snacks, but with more flexibility. So rather than your day going breakfast, lunch then snack, it's breakfast, snack and then a late lunch.

Your lunch might still get pushed back, but the overall structure and rhythm of your day stay much closer to normal. The outcome of that? Your energy is more stable, and so is your appetite.

Green flags!

The trifecta

This is a tool I use for busy social periods or travel, when routines are looser and it becomes harder to stick to your usual behaviours and rhythms.

We've all been there. You've got an event on, you don't eat beforehand and you tell yourself you will just grab something there. You arrive and go straight into a champagne or beer. The food you thought would be there is minimal or gets missed. You leave starving, swing past your favourite drive-through or kebab shop, get home later than normal, sleep in, skip your workout and start the next day with a greasy breakfast. Sound familiar?

So often, more drinks lead to poorer food choices, which then leads to less movement. That three-way slide is what I call the trifecta.

I first developed this framework in professional sport to help athletes navigate off-season periods so they could travel, switch off and still return meeting their fitness and body composition targets. I now use the same tool with people living busy, fast-paced lives or who travel regularly.

The trifecta has three parts: nutrition, exercise and alcohol. At any point, one of these can become more relaxed and it won't derail your rhythms or operating system too much. But if all three slip, your operating system is thrown into chaos.

Here's some examples of this in real life:

- If there are more drinks tonight, then tomorrow's exercise stays non-negotiable and your food choices remain as they normally do.
- If lunch is heavier and you want to have all three courses, then you don't drink, or you reduce your intake, and you stick to your exercise rhythm.
- If a workout is missed, then the nutrition stays dialled in and you skip the drinks.

The mistake many of us make in busy or social seasons is letting all three slip at once. More drinking, looser food choices and less movement—they compound, just not in the direction we want.

The trifecta works because it gives you structure that bends. It does not ask you to avoid life or stop having fun. It simply stops everything slipping at the same time, and best of all, you have complete decision-making power on what is going to work best for you on each occasion. It's another example of structured flexibility.

The one-day method

This is a tool for isolated occasions or celebrations, when one day has the potential to quickly turn into a week or a month. The end of the year is a common example of this. Calendars fill quickly, there are more social events, more food, more late nights and less routine.

In moments like this, I like to give people something simple to come back to. It is called the *one-day method*.

The idea is straightforward. Whatever you choose to eat, drink or do, it's just for one day. One day does not undo your foundations. The problem is not the day, the problem is when one day becomes a week, and a week becomes a month. That is when energy drops, sleep gets messy and your rhythms start to become undone.

This tool is about enjoying the day for what it is, then resetting and getting back to your usual behaviours, rhythms and operating system.

Get out of your own way

Once your operating system is in place, one of the biggest risks is sabotaging what's working, and getting in your own way.

This section sits alongside your daily operating system as a protective layer. It's for the moments when things are going well. You've made progress, you are being consistent and your daily operating system is working. You feel better, and yet a little voice starts to creep in and question whether it is enough.

This might show up as comparison, impatience, self-doubt or all-or-nothing thinking. If any of this sounds familiar, you are not alone. These are the moments where momentum can be sabotaged.

Here are three helpful reframes that help protect your progress if you notice this happening.

1. Progress over perfection

If I had a dollar for every time I said this line! This is the reframe you need when you start benchmarking against a past version of yourself, or the future version you think you should already be. It usually comes with a 'should' and it may sound like frustration and unrealistic expectations.

One of my favourite books, *The Gap and the Gain*, by Dan Sullivan and Benjamin Hardy, explains this well. The authors describe how many people measure themselves against the gap, the distance between where they are and where they think they should be. When you focus on the gap, dissatisfaction grows. You reinforce the idea that you are behind.

When you focus on the gain, you measure yourself against your past self. You look at how far you have come. That shift in behaviour and focus matters. It reinforces what is already working in your operating system, rather than pushing you to overhaul everything in the pursuit of perfection.

When you focus on the gap, dissatisfaction grows; when you focus on the gain, you see how far you have come.

So, next time you catch yourself in a comparison loop, or fixating on what is still missing, remind yourself that this is about progress, not perfection.

2. Sometimes a pause is the progress

This is another favourite saying of mine and one that is helpful when your operating system is working, your habits are consistent and you've made progress, but you hit a busy season, and life gets full or unpredictable.

In these moments, the win is not adding more, it is holding what you have already put in place. Especially if, in the past, this would have resulted in your behaviours and rhythms being inconsistent or stopping altogether.

When life gets busy, it is common for habits to slip and, soon after, energy drops, stress rises and recovery suffers. This is where a pause becomes progress. Holding your domino habit, protecting your non-negotiables and maintaining a scaled-back version of your usual rhythm is enough to keep your daily operating system intact. This is about stabilising, and stabilising during a demanding season, especially when habits would have slipped or stopped in the past, is progress.

3. How far ahead am I compared to before?

This is one I have started using more recently, and it tends to show up at a very specific point. You're on your health journey, living more aligned, proactive and intentionally. You've made progress, but the results you noticed earlier on, usually the external or objective ones, start to slow. And that's when the thought creeps in: *Nothing is happening.*

Here's an example of a conversation I had recently.

While building her company and raising her young family, Adela's health slowly moved to the bottom of her list of priorities in life. Over ten years of building her business, she gained about 25 to 30 kilos, barely exercised and became one of Uber Eats' best customers.

Eventually, she decided she wanted that to change. She started training a few times a week with a PT and walking daily. She had her bloods and key metrics done so she had baselines, and could see what impact her behaviour changes were having. She started planning meals and cooking more instead of ordering food. She stopped, or significantly reduced, drinking.

As a result, Adela lost 20 kilos, her biomarkers improved, and her energy was completely different. But then the external results, mainly her weight loss, slowed. Her focus shifted to how far she still wanted to go, instead of how far she had come.

In a conversation, I said to her, 'Think about how far you have come, and how far ahead you are compared to the past version of you.

Look at the decisions you are making and how you are moving through this summer, compared to even last year.'

This time around she was making sure she still had her delicious, satisfying breakfast, was exercising regularly and was keeping alcohol intake to a minimum. Previously, it would have looked very different. She would have slept in, exercise would not have been on the menu, and that would have been replaced with working through a cocktail list.

These decisions are compounding. Yes, more slowly now because the biggest upgrades have been made, and so much progress has already happened, but that does not mean they are not working and you need a new strategy. The operating system is doing its job. Green flags!

If you find yourself slipping back into the gap, or forgetting the progress you've made, here are some questions for you to reflect on to shift your focus and perspective.

- What am I doing consistently now that I wasn't doing six or 12 months ago?
- What behaviours that once required effort are now automatic?

Activity

It's time to bring everything together you've learnt throughout this book.

For each rhythm, write down the one behaviour you want to focus on now:

- Nutrition
- Exercise

(continued)

- Stress and recovery
- Sleep
- Connection.

Now look at this list and choose your top priority, where you want to start. Ask yourself, right now, what is my *domino habit*? What is the one habit that, when it's in place, makes everything else easier.

Lastly, identify your two to three *non-negotiables*. What are the habits you can commit to on your busiest days, not just your best.

This is the start of you building and sustaining your daily operating system.

Conclusion

As we get to the end, it's time to start building your daily operating system. It's time to reflect on where you are at, and think about the upgrades you might start to make, including what behaviours you'll implement (or stop), how the five rhythms work together, and how these will determine your energy, your capacity and recovery.

Your operating system is designed to work for your real life. In the weeks where things are predictable and structured, as well as in the weeks where plans change, demands increase and routine disappears. In those weeks, your operating system will provide you with structure and something to stabilise around.

Disruption does not mean you are off track. Travel, busy periods, illness, celebrations or unexpected events are part of life. Yes, they shift the conditions and context, but your operating system can bend and flex with that, allowing you structured flexibility.

Yes, this might mean scaling back to the bare minimum—your domino habit and non-negotiables. It might mean pausing rather than continuing to add (which is still progress). All of this is part of the system working as intended.

When you know how to anchor your days, adapt your rhythms and use simple tools to guide decisions under pressure or when self-sabotage creeps in, you can catch it and reframe it. This helps you see deviation not as disruption but as a gear shift that you have been equipped to manage.

This is how sustainable performance is created—through rhythms that support energy, capacity and recovery across changing seasons, rather than at the expense of them.

Your operating system is not something you complete or perfect, it is something you return to, refine and live with. The longer you work with it, the more intuitive it becomes and the easier it is to stay aligned, even when life gets full or messy.

And that is how sustainable success is achieved, because of wellbeing, not at its expense.

Not the end ... the beginning

While we may be at the end of our time together in this book, I hope that, for you, it really is just the beginning.

Some of you will read everything first, then come back and start implementing ideas. Some of you will have been making changes as you go. Others will read, reflect, pause and then decide what actually fits their life. However you have moved through these pages is exactly right for you.

My intention with this book was simple: to make complex science practical, relatable and easy to use. For too long, health has been made to feel hard, overwhelming and like it requires a complete overhaul of your life. It doesn't.

Spending more than 15 years deep in this world, working with thousands of people, has given me a very clear view. I see the patterns, what sticks and the blind spots. And I see how small, intentional changes can quietly but powerfully change the entire direction of your life.

But this book is not only shaped by my professional experience. It has also been shaped by my own journey—from those early days in the pool, through periods of intensity, imbalance and learning things the hard way. I am not someone who just teaches this work, I am someone who has lived it and often had to relearn it. Those experiences are why this book exists.

Everything in these pages has been designed to follow the architecture of your day. From how you start, to how you move through it, to how you recover from it. Health touches every part of your life. It is truly complex by nature, but it does not need to be complicated. My goal is to give you direction without rigidity, a framework without perfection, structure with flexibility.

This is about building a version of life that suits you. This book is not meant to just sit on a shelf once you have finished reading. Hopefully, you will return to it, dip back into it, and revisit it as life changes, seasons shift and priorities evolve.

Health is the foundation of performance. It is also the thing we most easily take for granted until it is compromised. I love this saying: *a healthy person has a thousand goals, an unhealthy person has one.* It's true. Health is our greatest wealth!

There are not many things in life that are a 24-7 process, but health is one of them. This is why we must move away from binary thinking. Away from all-or-nothing approaches. Away from the belief that a lifetime of habits can be fixed with a six-week challenge or a burst of motivation. Health does not require perfection, it requires consistency and adaptability.

Yes, what you eat matters. How you move your body matters. How you manage stress and recovery matters. How you sleep matters. But so does your purpose, your values and how connected you are to them and to the people around you. Sustainable performance is not built in isolation.

This book was written with two things in mind: helping you feel better in your real life, right now, and supporting the future version of you. When you have big, audacious goals, it is easy for health to slip down the priority list. But when you prioritise health (and yourself), it becomes the foundation that helps you not just survive demanding seasons, but thrive in them.

If you do nothing else after this book, choose one small thing you want to change and start there. If I can give you one final prompt, think about your domino habit: the one behaviour that sets the tone for everything else that follows. Identify it, protect it, return to it. Let it anchor your daily operating system.

This is not about becoming someone new or overhauling your current behaviours, it is about upgrading or adding to what you're currently doing to give you more energy, help you recover better and to achieve sustainable performance in a way that works for you now, and in the future too.

Jess x

PS: If this work has resonated, I would love to stay connected. You can find me on LinkedIn and Instagram, where I share more of this thinking and my insights. I also host a podcast called *Stay at the Top*, where I explore these ideas through solo episodes and conversations with leaders, elite athletes and other health performance experts — covering the science, systems and practical strategies behind sustainable success.

If you want to bring this work to your people, team or organisation, this is what I do and love. Through keynotes, workshops, programs and advisory work, all focused on turning wellbeing into your performance edge. Use the QR code below or go to jessicaspendlove.com for more information.

Acknowledgements

The idea of writing a book sat with me for many years. It always felt like something I would get around to when the time was right, or when I finally had the time. After several conversations with different people and publishing houses over the years, I realised there is no such thing as the perfect time. There is only the mission, the impact you want to create, and the decision to make time for what matters.

In many ways, this book reflects the very principles I speak about in my work. Sustainable performance is not about waiting for ideal conditions, it is about prioritising what matters and creating the space for it.

When the idea of writing a book first emerged, it was going to be a nutrition book. That made sense, given nutrition is where I have spent most of my career. But, over time, I felt a pull in a different direction to a broader conversation that sits at the intersection of wellbeing and high performance. Nutrition is a critical piece of that puzzle, but it is only one part of the system that allows people to perform well and sustain success over time.

Being science trained, with two degrees and the beginning of a PhD that I never finished, I have always been curious about where the evidence sits and how different disciplines intersect. Over the past few years, this work has come to life through my keynotes, workshops and programs, and this book is a continuation of that journey.

While writing a book felt like something I was meant to do, there was also doubt. At school, maths and science were my stronger subjects and English required a little more work. Most of what I had written in the course of my career was in a very different format to a book. But, over time, refining my thinking, strengthening my message and recognising the mission behind the work made it clear that this book needed to exist.

After years of thinking about it, a few fruitful conversations and the opportunity to publish within a short timeline, the wheels were finally set in motion. I also did this while raising a one-year-old. I used to imagine writing a book would be done somewhere remote and locking myself away to focus entirely on the manuscript. Instead, it was written between early mornings, longer days and weekends. As I often say, you make time for what matters.

Firstly, to myself. For believing I could do it in this season of life. I could have found every excuse as to why now was not the time. But after spending years thinking through what my message and book would be, seeing how my lived personal and professional experience could make a difference, and remembering the many times I got it wrong—when I ran myself into the ground and let ambition come close to costing me the most important thing, my health—I knew it was time. This is something I see in so many motivated and driven people. It was not about finding time. It was about making time.

To my partner Sam and my angel Millie, thank you. Navigating motherhood, running a business and writing a book is not something you do alone. Writing this meant early starts, longer days and weekends at the laptop, and that was only possible because Sam stepped up even more to help with Millie during that time. If I ever write another book, I might finally test the idea of disappearing to the countryside or a quiet island to write it.

To the people who helped me believe there was a book in me. Julie Mazur Tribe, who first reached out and made me think I had a book in me. Thank you for your belief and the connection we have built over the years. Glen James, who I ran into at SXSW Sydney and who became the catalyst. That conversation ultimately led to my introduction to Lucy Raymond at Wiley, which is where this book found its home.

To the entire Wiley team, thank you for making this process collaborative, thoughtful and genuinely enjoyable. Your support helped me crystallise my ideas, refine the message and shape this work into something that could live in the world. In particular, thank you to Lucy, Leigh, Ingrid and Melanie.

To the unconditional friendships in my life that remain constant regardless of time, distance or busy seasons. Thank you for always being there, and for understanding that even when life gets full, those connections remain.

To my parents, thank you for always supporting my dreams. From waking up at 4 am to drive me across Sydney for swimming training, to providing every kind of emotional and practical support along the way. On a side note, I hope Millie does not decide she wants to become a national-level swimmer. I am not sure I am ready for those early mornings again!

And, finally, to my clients. The athletes, leaders and teams I have had the privilege of working with over the past 15 years. Your curiosity, commitment and pursuit of excellence have shaped so much of what lives inside this book. The lessons in these pages are not theoretical. They are drawn from the real challenges and conversations we have shared together. Thank you for trusting me to be part of your journey.

And finally, to you, the reader. Thank you for your interest in my work. If you are reading this book, I know you care about improving yourself and the life you are building. My guess is that you have spent a lot of your time and energy focused on your career, your business or your ambitions. But, as I have learnt, there is so much more to life than that, and wellbeing is the foundation of everything. I hope this book helps you prioritise yourself, something that can be surprisingly difficult to do. The upside is that when you do, not only do you benefit, but so does everyone around you.

References

1. Corporate Mental Health Alliance Australia 2025, 'The leading mentally healthy workplaces survey reports', Corporate Mental Health AllianceAustralia, https://cmhaa.org.au/wp-content/uploads/CMHAA-Survey-Report-2025_digital_Final.pdf.
2. Beyond Blue 2025, '1 in 2 Australians facing workplace burnout', Beyond Blue, https://www.beyondblue.org.au/about/media/media-releases/1-in-2-Australians-Facing-Workplace-Burnout.
3. Harrell, E 2015, '1% performance improvements led to Olympic gold', *Harvard Business Review*,https://hbr.org/2015/10/how-1-performance-improvements-led-to-olympic-gold.
4. Clear, J 2018, *Atomic Habits: An easy and proven way to build good habits and break bad ones*, Avery Pub Group.
5. Spendlove, JK, Heaney, SE, Gifford, JA, et al. 2012, 'Evaluation of general nutrition knowledge in elite Australian athletes', *British Journal of Nutrition*, vol. 107, no. 12, pp. 1871–80.
6. Schwartz, T, McCarthy, C 2007, 'Manage your energy, not your time', *Harvard Business Review*, https://hbr.org/2007/10/manage-your-energy-not-your-time.
7. Loehr, J, Schwartz, T 2003, *The Power of Full Engagement: Managing energy, not time, is the key to high performance and personal renewal*, New York: Free Press.
8. Cepni, AB, Kirschmann, JM, Rodriguezm A, et al. 2025, 'When routines break: The health implications of disrupted daily life', *American Journal of Lifestyle Medicine*, 15598276251381626. [online ahead of print].
9. Sustainability Directory n.d., 'What is the role of routine in mitigating decisionfatigue?', https://lifestyle.sustainability-directory.com/learn/what-is-the-role-of-routine-in-mitigating-decision-fatigue/.

10. Work Well Leaders 2025, 'WorkWell Leaders impact measure and roadmap: Groundbreaking study finds leader wellbeing has the most significant impact on organisational wellbeing and performance', Work Well Leaders, https://www.workwellleaders.org/programmes/work well-leaders-impact-measure/.
11. Walker, M 2017, *Why We Sleep: Unlocking the power of sleep and dreams,* Penguin Random House.
12. *Huberman Lab* 2025, Boost your energy and immune system with cortisol and adrenaline, YouTube, https://www.youtube.com/watch?v=wFucddupQlk.
13. Wiłkość-Dębczyńska, M, Liberacka-Dwojak, M 2023, 'Time of day and chronotype in the assessment of cognitive functions', *Postępy Psychiatrii i Neurologii*, vol. 32, no. 3, pp. 162–6.
14. Breus, M 2016, *The Power of When: Discover your chronotype—and the best time to eat lunch, ask for a raise, have sex, write a novel, take your meds, and more,* Little, Brown Spark.
15. Sharma, R 2018, *The 5 AM Club: Own your morning. Elevate your life,* HarperCollins Publishers.
16. Shaheen, A, Sadiya, A, Mussa, BM, et al. 2024, 'Postprandial glucose and insulin response to meal sequence among healthy UAE adults: a randomised controlled crossover trial', *Diabetes, Metabolic Syndrome and Obesity*, vol. 17, pp. 4257–65.
17. Bermingham, KM, May, A, Asnicar, F, et al. 2023, 'Snack quality and snack timing are associated with cardiometabolic blood markers: The ZOE PREDICT study', *European Journal of Nutrition*, vol. 63, no. 1, pp. 121–3.
18. Adams, J 2024, 'The NOVA system can be used to address harmful foods and harmful food systems', *PLoS Medicine*, vol. 21, no. 11, p. e1004492.
19. Machado, PP, Steele, EM, Levy, RB, et al. 2020, 'Ultra-processed food consumption and obesity in the Australian adult population', *Nutrition and Diabetes*, vol. 10, no. 1, p. 39.
20. Lane, MM, Gamage, E, Du, S, et al. 2024, 'Ultra-processed food exposure and adverse health outcomes: Umbrella review of epidemiological meta-analyses', *BMJ*, vol. 384, p. e077310.
21. Areta, JL, Burke, LM, Ross, ML, et al. 2013, 'Timing and distribution of protein ingestion during prolonged recovery from resistance exercise alters myofibrillar protein synthesis', *The Journal of Physiology*, vol. 591, no. 9, pp. 2319–31.

22. Nunes, EA, Colenso-Semple, L, McKellar, SR 2022, 'Systematic review and meta-analysis of protein intake to support muscle mass and function in healthy adults', *Journal of Cachexia, Sarcopenia and Muscle*, vol. 13, no. 2, pp. 795–810.
23. Cruz-Jentoft, AJ, Sayer, AA 2019, 'Sarcopenia', *The Lancet*, vol. 393, no. 10191, pp. 2636–46.
24. Drummen, M, Tischmann, L, Gatta-Cherifi, B, et al. 2018, 'Dietary protein and energy balance in relation to obesity and co-morbidities', *Frontiers in Endocrinology*, vol. 9, p. 443.
25. Leidy, HJ, Racki, EM 2010, 'The addition of a protein-rich breakfast and its effects on acute appetite control and food intake in breakfast-skipping adolescents', *International Journal of Obesity*, vol. 34, no. 7, pp. 1125–33.
26. Williamson, E, Moore, DR 2021, 'A muscle-centric perspective on intermittent fasting: A suboptimal dietary strategy for supporting muscle protein remodeling and muscle mass?', *Frontiers in Nutrition*, vol. 8, p. 640621.
27. Zeb, F, Osaili, T, Obaid, RS, et al. 2023, 'Gut microbiota and time-restricted feeding/eating: A targeted biomarker and approach in precision nutrition', *Nutrients*, vol. 15, no. 2, p. 259.
28. McDonald, D, Hyde, E, Debelius, JW, et al. 2018, 'American gut: An open platform for citizen science microbiome research', *mSystems*, vol. 3, no. 3, pp. e00031-18.
29. Wiertsema, SP, van Bergenhenegouwen, J, Garssen, J, et al. 2021, 'The interplay between the gut microbiome and the immune system in the context of infectious diseases throughout life and the role of nutrition in optimising treatment strategies', *Nutrients*, vol. 13, no. 3, p. 886.
30. Rossi, M, Johnson, AJ, Nelson, AM, et al. 2019, 'Gut microbiota composition and nutrient intake are associated with wellbeing in a population-based cohort', *BMJ Open*, vol. 9, p. e026845.
31. Chen, Y, Xu, J, Chen, Y 2021, 'Regulation of neurotransmitters by the gut microbiota and effects on cognition in neurological disorders', *Nutrients*, vol. 13, no. 6, p. 2099.
32. Bonaz, B, Bazin, T, Pellissier, S 2018, 'The vagus nerve at the interface of the microbiota-gut-brain axis', *Frontiers in Neuroscience*, vol. 12, p. 49.
33. Van Oudenhove, L, Crowell, MD, Drossman, DA, et al. 2016, 'Biopsychosocial aspects of functional gastrointestinal disorders', *Gastroenterology*, vol. S0016-5085, no. 16, pp. 00218-3.

34. Hetta, HF, Sirag, N, Elfadil, H, et al. 2023, 'Artificial sweeteners: A double-edged sword for gut microbiome', *Diseases*, vol. 13, no. 4, p. 115.
35. Dmytriv, TR, Storey, KB, Lushchak, VI 2024, 'Intestinal barrier permeability: The influence of gut microbiota, nutrition, and exercise', *Frontiers in Physiology*, vol. 15, p. 1380713.
36. Di Vincenzo, F, Del Gaudio, A, Petito, V 2023, 'Gut microbiota, intestinal permeability, and systemic inflammation: A narrative review', *Internal and Emergency Medicine*, vol. 19, no. 2, pp. 275–93.
37. Burke, LM, Hawley, JA, Wong, SH, et al. 2011, 'Carbohydrates for training and competition', *Journal of Sports Science*, vol. 29, Suppl 1, pp. S17–27.
38. Adan, A 2012 'Cognitive performance and dehydration', *Journal of the American College of Nutrition*, vol. 31, no. 2, pp. 71–8.
39. Upadhyay, M, McNeil-Masuka, J, Srinivas, V 2023, *Insensible fluid loss*, StatPearls Publishing, https://www.ncbi.nlm.nih.gov/books/NBK544219.
40. WHOOP, 'How digestion and fasting impact sleep quality and consistency', WHOOP, https://www.whoop.com/au/en/thelocker/promoting-digestion-to-improve-sleep/.
41. Barker, L, Cawley, A, Speers, N, et al. 2025, 'Sports supplement analysis survey for the prevalence of WADA prohibited substances in the Australian online marketplace', *Drug Testing and Analysis*, no. 17, no. 10, pp. 1857–64.
42. Sjöblom, L, Bonn, SE, Alexandrou, C, et al., 2023, 'Dietary habits after a physical activity mHealth intervention: A randomised controlled trial', *BMC Nutrition*, vol 9, no 1, p. 23.
43. Basso, JC, Suzuki, WA 2017, 'The effects of acute exercise on mood, cognition, neurophysiology, and neurochemical pathways: A review', *Brain Plasticity*, vol. 2, no. 2, pp. 127–52.
44. Lang, JJ, Prince, SA, Merucci,K, et al. 2021, 'Cardiorespiratory fitness is a strong and consistent predictor of morbidity and mortality among adults: An overview of meta-analyses representing over 20.9 million observations from 199 unique cohort studies', *British Journal of Sports Medicine*, vol, 55, no. 21, pp. 1199–205.
45. Shi, Y, Zhang, Y, Yang, X, et al. 2025, 'The relationship between cognitive function and muscle mass in older adults: A longitudinal study based on CLHLS', *Frontiers in Psychiatry*, vol. 16, p. 1595625.
46. Momma, H, Kawakami, R, Honda, T, et al. 2022, 'Muscle-strengthening activities are associated with lower risk and mortality in major

non-communicable diseases: A systematic review and meta-analysis of cohort studies', *British Journal of Sports Medicine,* vol. 56, no. 13, pp. 755–63.

47. Kagendo, JI, Watson, B 2026, 'Resistance training to mitigate sarcopenia in menopausal women', *Research in Sport Performance,* vol. 6, no. 1, pp. 1–4.
48. American College of Sports Medicine 2009, 'Progression models in resistance training for healthy adults', *Medicine and Science in Sports and Exercise,* vol. 41, no. 3, pp. 687–708.
49. Wilkinson, DJ, Piasecki, M, Atherton, PJ 2018, 'The age-related loss of skeletal muscle mass and function: Measurement and physiology of muscle fibre atrophy and muscle fibre loss in humans', *Ageing Research Reviews,* vol. 47, pp. 123–32.
50. Karlamangla, AS, Burnett-Bowie, SM, Crandall, CJ 2018, 'Bone health during the menopause transition and beyond', *Obstetrics and Gynecology Clinics of North America,* vol. 45, no. 4, pp. 695–708.
51. Stamatakis, E, Biswas, RK, Koemel, NA 2025, 'Dose response of incidental physical activity against cardiovascular events and mortality', *Circulation,* vol. 151, no. 15.
52. Department of Health, Disability and Ageing 2021, 'Physical activity and exercise guidelines for all Australians', Australian Government, https://www.health.gov.au/topics/physical-activity-and-exercise/physical-activity-and-exercise-guidelines-for-all-australians.
53. Alexe, DI, Saha, S, Choudhary, PK 2025, 'Exercise snacks as a strategy to interrupt sedentary behavior: A systematic review of health outcomes and feasibility', *Healthcare (Basel),* vol. 13, no. 24, p. 3216.
54. Chen, J, Lu, Y, Zhao, H, et al. 2025, 'The effectiveness of exercise snacks as a time-efficient treatment for improving cardiometabolic health in adults: A systematic review and meta-analysis', *Frontiers in Cardiovascular Medicine,* vol. 12, p. 1643153.
55. Attia, P 2025, 'Your grip strength could predict your lifespan', YouTube, https://www.youtube.com/shorts/YulI5lspQWk.
56. Paluch, AE, Bajpai, S, Bassett, DR, et al. 2021, 'Daily steps and all-cause mortality in middle-aged adults in the coronary artery risk development in young adults study', *JAMA Network Open,* vol. 4, no. 9, p. e2124516.
57. Aird, TP, Davies, RW, Carson, BP 2018, 'Effects of fasted vs fed-state exercise on performance and post-exercise metabolism: A systematic review and meta-analysis', *Scandinavian Journal of Medicine and Science in Sports,* vol. 28, no. 5, pp. 1476–90.

58. Headspace 2025, 'Nearly half of young Australians experiencing high levels of psychological distress—but more are seeking support', Headspace, https://headspace.org.au/our-organisation/media-releases/nearly-half-of-young-australians-experiencing-high-levels-of-psychological-distress-but-more-are-seeking-support.
59. Allianz 2025, 'Australian employees call for structural change amid mental distress in the workplace', Allianz, https://www.allianz.com.au/about-us/media-hub/structural-change-amid-workplace-mental-distress.html.
60. Hosie, R 2025, 'Novak Djokovic is winning titles at 38. He credits his longevity to 3 simple things', *Business Insider*, https://www.businessinsider.com/changes-novak-djokovic-tennis-longevity-diet-sleep-emotional-health-2025-11.
61. Uphill, A, Kendall, KL, Guppy, S, et al. 2021, 'Neuromuscular performance changes in response to the Australian Special Forces selection course', *Journal of Science and Medicine in Sport*, vol. 24, no. 8, pp. 781–6.
62. Guidi, J, Lucente, M, Sonino, N, et al. 2021, 'Allostatic load and its impact on health: A systematic review', *Psychotherapy and Psychosomatics*, vol. 90, no. 1, pp. 11–27.
63. Castellani, JW, Young, AJ 2016, 'Human physiological responses to cold exposure: Acute responses and acclimatization to prolonged exposure', *Autonomic Neuroscience: Basic and Clinical*, vol. 196, pp. 63–74.
64. Cain, T, Brinsley, J, Bennett, H, et al. 2025, 'Effects of cold-water immersion on health and wellbeing: A systematic review and meta-analysis', *PLoS One*, vol. 20, no. 1, p. e0317615.
65. Laukkanen, T, Kunutsor, SK, Khan, H, et al. 2018, 'Sauna bathing is associated with reduced cardiovascular mortality and improves risk prediction in men and women: A prospective cohort study', *BMC Medicine*, vol. 16, no. 1, p. 219.
66. Lee, EM, Kolunsarka, IA, Kostensalo, J, et al. 2022, 'Effects of regular sauna bathing in conjunction with exercise on cardiovascular function: A multi-arm randomized controlled trial', *American Journal of Physiology-Regulatory, Integrative and Comparative Physiology*, vol. 323, no. 3, pp. R289–99.
67. Laukkanen, T, Lipponen, J, Kunutsor, SK, et al. 2019, 'Recovery from sauna bathing favorably modulates cardiac autonomic nervous system', *Complementary Therapies in Medicine*, vol. 45, pp. 190–7.

68. Haghayegh, S, Khoshnevis, S, Smolensky, MH, et al. 2019, 'Before-bedtime passive body heating by warm shower or bath to improve sleep: A systematic review and meta-analysis', *Sleep Medicine Reviews*, vol. 46, pp. 124–35.
69. Laukkanen, JA, Laukkanen, T, Kunutsor, SK 2018, 'Cardiovascular and other health benefits of sauna bathing: A review of the evidence', *Mayo Clinic Proceedings*, vol. 93, no. 8, pp. 1111–21.
70. Fraser, A 2014, *The Third Space: Using life's little transitions to find balance and happiness*, Random House Australia.
71. Albulescu, P, Macsinga, I, Rusu, A, et al. 2022, 'Give me a break! A systematic review and meta-analysis on the efficacy of micro-breaks for increasing well-being and performance', *PLoS One*, vol. 17, no. 8, p. e0272460.
72. White, MP, Elliott, LR, Grellier, J, et al. 2021, 'Associations between green/blue spaces and mental health across 18 countries', *Scientific Reports*, vol. 11, p. 8903.
73. Olszewska-Guizzo, A, Sia, A, Fogel, A, et al. 2022, 'Features of urban green spaces associated with positive emotions, mindfulness and relaxation', *Scientific Reports*, vol. 12, p. 20388.
74. Sonnentag, S 2012, 'Psychological detachment from work during leisure time: The benefits of mentally disengaging from work', *Current Directions in Psychological Science*, vol. 21, no. 2, pp. 114–8.
75. Syrek, CJ, de Bloom, J, Lehr, D 2021, 'Well recovered and more creative? A longitudinal study on the relationship between vacation and creativity', *Frontiers in Psychology*, vol. 12, p. 784844.
76. Blank, C, Gatterer, K, Leichtfried, V, et al. 2018, 'Short vacation improves stress level and well-being in German-speaking middle-managers: A randomised controlled trial', *International Journal of Environmental Research and Public Health*, vol. 15, no. 1, p. 130.
77. Nawijn, J, Marchand, MA, Veenhoven, R, et al. 2010, 'Vacationers happier, but most not happier after a holiday', *Applied Research in Quality of Life*, vol. 5, no. 1, pp. 35–47.
78. Sleep Health n.d. 'Chronic insomnia disorder in Australia', Sleep Health, https://www.sleephealthfoundation.org.au/special-sleep-reports/chronic-insomnia-disorder-in-australia.
79. Chaput, J-P, Dutil, C, Featherstone, R, et al. 2020, 'Sleep timing, sleep consistency, and health in adults: A systematic review', *Applied Physiology, Nutrition and Metabolism*, vol. 45, no. 10, Suppl 2, p. S232–S247.

80. Zuraikat, FM, Makarem N, Redline S, et al. 2020, 'Sleep regularity and cardiometabolic health: Is variability in sleep patterns a risk factor for excess adiposity and glycaemic dysregulation?', *Current Diabetes Reports,* vol. 20, no. 8, p. 38.
81. Reytor-González, C, Simancas-Racines, D, Román-Galeano, NM, et al. 2025, 'Chrononutrition and energy balance: How meal timing and circadian rhythms shape weight regulation and metabolic health', *Nutrients*, vol. 17, no. 13, p. 2135.
82. WHOOP 2023, 'How digestion and fasting impact sleep quality and consistency', WHOOP, https://www.whoop.com/au/en/thelocker/promoting-digestion-to-improve-sleep/.
83. Leota, J, Presby, DM, Le, F, et al. 2025, 'Dose-response relationship between evening exercise and sleep/autonomic activity: A large-scale wearable sensor cohort study', *Nature Communications*, vol. 16, p. 2486.
84. Gardiner, C, Weakley, J, Burke, LM, et al. 2023, 'The effect of caffeine on subsequent sleep: A systematic review and meta-analysis', *Sleep Medicine Reviews*, vol. 69, p. 101764.
85. Mograss, M, Abi-Jaoude, J, Frimpong, E, et al. 2022, 'The effects of napping on night-time sleep in healthy young adults', *Journal of Sleep Research,* vol. 31, no. 5, p. e13578.
86. Centofanti, S, Banks, S, Coussens, S, et al. 2020, 'A pilot study investigating the impact of a caffeine-nap on alertness during a simulated night shift', *Chronobiology International*, vol. 37, no. 9–10, pp. 1469–73.
87. ACP Newsroom 2016, 'ACP recommends cognitive behavioral therapy as initial treatment for chronic insomnia', ACP Newsroom, https://www.acponline.org/acp-newsroom/acp-recommends-cognitive-behavioral-therapy-as-initial-treatment-forchronic-insomnia.
88. Mayo Clinic n.d., Obstructive sleep apnea, Mayo Clinic, https://www.mayoclinic.org/diseases-conditions/obstructive-sleep-apnea/symptoms-causes/syc-20352090.
89. Cleveland Clinic 2023, Restless legs syndrome, Cleveland Clinic, https://my.clevelandclinic.org/health/diseases/9497-restless-legs-syndrome.
90. Greer, SM, Goldstein, AN, Walker, MP 2013, 'The impact of sleep deprivation on food desire in the human brain', *Nature Communications*, vol. 4, p. 2259.
91. Hausenblas, HA, Lynch, T, Hooper, S, et al. 2024, 'Magnesium-L-threonate improves sleep quality and daytime functioning in adults with self-reported sleep problems: A randomised controlled trial', *Sleep Medicine: X*, vol. 8, p. 100121.

92. Schuster, J, Cycelskij, I, Lopresti, A, et al. 2025, 'Magnesium bisglycinate supplementation in healthy adults reporting poor sleep: A randomized, placebo-controlled trial', *Nature and Science of Sleep*, vol. 17, pp. 2027–40.
93. Losso, JN, Finley, JW, Karki, N, et al. 2018, 'Pilot study of the tart cherry juice for the treatment of insomnia and investigation of mechanisms', *American Journal of Therapeutics*, vol. 25, no. 4, pp. e680–e686.
94. Howatson, G, Bell, PG, Tallent, J, et al. 2012, 'Effect of tart cherry juice (*Prunus cerasus*) on melatonin levels and enhanced sleep quality', *European Journal of Nutrition*, vol. 51, no. 8, pp. 909–16.
95. Vitale, KC, Hueglin, S, Broad, EM 2017, 'Tart cherry juice in athletes: A literature review and commentary', *Current Sports Medicine Reports*, vol. 16, no. 4, pp. 230–9.
96. Zick, SM, Wright, BD, Sen, A, et al. 2011, 'Preliminary examination of the efficacy and safety of a standardized chamomile extract for chronic primary insomnia: A randomized placebo-controlled pilot trial', *BMC Complementary and Alternative Medicine*, vol. 11, p. 78.
97. Gordji-Nejad, A, Matusch, A, Kleedörfer, S, et al. 2024, 'Single dose creatine improves cognitive performance and induces changes in cerebral high energy phosphates during sleep deprivation', *Scientific Reports*, vol. 14, p. 4937.
98. Candow, DG, Forbes, SC, Ostojic, SM, et al. 2023, '"Heads Up" for creatine supplementation and its potential applications for brain health and function', *Sports Medicine*, vol. 53, suppl 1, pp. 49–65.
99. Cacioppo, JT, Cacioppo, S, Capitanio, JP, et al. 2014, 'The neuroendocrinology of social isolation', *Annual Review of Psychology*, vol. 66, pp. 733–67.
100. Holt-Lunstad, J, Smith, TB, Layton, JB 2010, 'Social relationships and mortality risk: A meta-analytic review', *PLoS Medicine*, vol. 7, no. 7, p. e1000316.
101. World Health Organization n.d., WHO commission on social connection, WHO, https://www.who.int/groups/commission-on-social-connection.
102. Eisenberger, NI, Lieberman, MD 2004, 'Why rejection hurts: A common neural alarm system for physical and social pain', *Trends in Cognitive Sciences*, vol. 8, no. 7, pp. 294–300.
103. Alimujiang, A, Wiensch, A, Boss, J, et al. 2019, 'Association between life purpose and mortality among US adults older than 50 years', *JAMA Network Open*, vol. 2, no. 5, p. e194270.

104. Buettner, D, Skemp, S 2016, 'Blue Zones: Lessons from the world's longest lived', *American Journal of Lifestyle Medicine*, vol. 10, no. 5, pp. 318–21.
105. Hostinar, CE, Gunnar, MR 2015, 'Social support can buffer against stress and shape brain activity', *AJOB Neuroscience*, vol. 6, no. 3, pp. 34–42.
106. Gunnar, MR, Hostinar, CE 2015, 'The social buffering of the hypothalamic–pituitary–adrenocortical axis in humans: Developmental and experiential determinants', *Social Neuroscience*, vol. 10, no. 5, pp. 479–88.
107. Milyavskaya, M, Galla, BM, Inzlicht, M, et al. 2021, 'More effort, less fatigue: The role of interest in increasing effort and reducing mental fatigue', *Frontiers in Psychology*, vol. 12, p. 755858.
108. Boehm, JK 2021, 'Positive psychological well-being and cardiovascular disease: Exploring mechanistic and developmental pathways', *Social and Personality Psychology Compass*, vol. 15, no. 6, p. e12599.
109. Mineo, L 2017, 'Good genes are nice, but joy is better', *The Harvard Gazette*, https://news.harvard.edu/gazette/story/2017/04/over-nearly-80-years-harvard-study-has-been-showing-how-to-live-a-healthy-and-happy-life/.
110. Waldinger, R, 2016, 'What makes a good life? Lessons from the longest study on happiness', YouTube, https://www.youtube.com/watch?v=8KkKuTCFvzI.
111. Allen, K-A, Kern, ML, Rozek, CS, et al. 2021, 'Belonging: A review of conceptual issues, an integrative framework, and directions for future research', *Australian Journal of Psychology*, vol. 73, no. 1, pp. 87–102.
112. Blom, V 2012, 'Contingent self-esteem, stressors and burnout in working women and men', *Work*, vol. 43, no. 2, pp. 123–31.
113. Figueiredo, E, Margaça, C, Sánchez-García, JC 2025, 'Loneliness and isolation in the era of telework: A comprehensive review of challenges for organizational success, *Healthcare*, vol. 13, no. 16, p. 1943.
114. Korkmaz, U, Şimşek, MH, Şahin, ÖF 2025, 'The effect of emotion regulation difficulties and loneliness on anxiety, depression, and stress levels in remote workers', *BMC Public Health*, vol. 25, p. 2572.
115. Stieger, S, Lewetz, D, Willinger, D 2023, 'Face-to-face more important than digital communication for mental health during the pandemic', *Scientific Reports*, vol. 13, p. 802.

116. Akash, MS, Chowdhury, S 2025, 'Small changes, big impact: A mini review of habit formation and behavioral change principles', *World Journal of Advanced Research and Reviews*, vol. 26, no. 1, pp. 3098–106.
117. Gardner, B, Lally, P, Wardle, J 2012, 'Making health habitual: The psychology of "habit formation" and general practice', *British Journal of General Practice*, vol. 62, no. 605, pp. 664–6.
118. Singh, B, Murphy, A, Maher, C 2024, 'Time to form a habit: A systematic review and meta-analysis of health behaviour habit formation and its determinants', *Healthcare (Basel)*, vol. 12, no. 23, p. 2488.

Printed and bound by CPI Group (UK) Ltd, Croydon, CR0 4YY

20/07/2026

14925137-0001